What This Book Is About. . . .

When Tom Warren was diagnosed as having Alzheimer's disease, neither he, a successful insurance agent, nor his wife, a practicing pharmacologist, accepted the doctor's finding as final. While no one had ever documented a reversal of Alzheimer's, they refused to believe there was nothing they could do. For six years, Tom — during his lucid periods — and his wife pored through all the medical literature, both orthodox and alternative. What they found, as astonishing as it sounds, was enough information for Tom Warren to develop an effective treatment that would beat his "incurable" disease.

Beating Alzheimer's is the true story of Tom Warren and his experience with Alzheimer's disease. In it, Tom outlines the step-by-step plan that he followed to free himself from the grips of this relentless disease. Tom includes the latest documented research that explains why his treatment worked, and why it may also work for other related brain diseases.

Although this nontoxic, noninvasive treatment is relatively new, as word has spread, many physicians have contacted Tom and have put their patients on his program with very positive results. This book makes this plan directly available to the general public for the first time.

BEATING ALZHEIMER'S

A STEP TOWARDS UNLOCKING
THE MYSTERIES OF BRAIN DISEASES

TOM WARREN

AVERY
a member of Penguin Putnam Inc.

The diet and health procedures in this book are based on the personal experiences of the author. Because each person and situation are unique, the editor and the publisher urge the reader to check with a qualified health professional before using any procedure where there is any question concerning appropriateness. The publisher does not advocate the use of any particular diet or treatment, but believes the information presented in this book should be available to the public. Because there is always some risk involved, the author and publisher are not responsible for any adverse effects or consequences from the use of any of the suggestions in this book. Please do not use the suggestions in this book if you are unwilling to assume the risk. Feel free to consult a physician or other qualified health professional. It is a sign of wisdom, not cowardice, to seek a second or third opinion.

Cover design: Rudy Shur and Janine Eisner-Wall
In-house editor: Elaine Will Sparber
Typesetting: Coghill Book Typesetting Company, Richmond, Virginia

Library of Congress Cataloging-in-Publication Data

Warren, Tom.
   Beating Alzheimer's : a step towards unlocking the mysteries of brain disease / Tom Warren.
     p. cm.
   Includes bibliographical references and index.
   ISBN 0-89529-488-5 (quality pbk.)
   1. Alzheimer's disease—Treatment—Case studies. I. Title.
   [DNLM: 1. Alzheimer's Disease—therapy—personal narratives. WM 220 W293b]
RC523.W37 1991
616.8'3106—dc20
DNLM/DLC
for Library of Congress   91-17211
                                CIP

Printed in the United States of America.

20 19 18 17 16 15

Contents

To my wife, Louise, who loved me and supported me, and without whose help I would have died years ago.

With special remembrance, posthumously, to Father Allen Amirault—"Boston Blackie"—former chaplain, psychologist, professor, and friend, who said, "There is something we do not understand about mental illness. We think people are a lot more responsible for their actions than they actually are."

The excerpt on pages 28-29 is reprinted with the permission of Sam Ziff, publisher and editor, *Bio-Probe* magazine.

The advertisement on page 61 is reprinted with the permission of the Skagit County Public Utility District.

The table on pages 74-78 is used with the permission of Avery Publishing Group. It was adapted from *The Real Vitamin and Mineral Book: Going Beyond the RDA for Optimum Health* © 1990 by Shari Lieberman and Nancy Bruning.

The excerpt on page 103 is reprinted with the permission of Dr. Russell Jaffe, director, Princeton BioCenter.

The PAR Booklet, © 1989 by Huggins Diagnostic Inc., reprinted in Appendix E, is used with the permission of Dr. Hal A. Huggins.

Acknowledgments

I call *Beating Alzheimer's* my story, but that is not accurate. The credit for both my recovery and book belongs to more than just me—my wife, Louise; the Well Mind Association, of Seattle, Washington; some of the best physicians in the world; and, of course, God's blessings and mercy.

Many thanks must also go to the allergy patients, the physicians, and the other medical professionals who read my manuscript and made many thoughtful suggestions. To Sandra Denton, M.D.; Richard Wilkinson, M.D.; Russell Jaffe, M.D.; William G. Crook, M.D.; Abram Hoffer, M.D.; Hal Huggins, D.D.S.; Sam Ziff and his son, Michael Ziff, D.D.S.; and the authors of the numerous books and medical reports I read that literally saved my life: Thank you.

I would also like to thank Susan Carskadon, my agent, who made many thoughtful suggestions that are now a part of the book.

Other wonderful, helpful people edited my manuscript over the several years that this work has been in progress. To each and every one of them, my heartfelt thanks. Because of your selfless efforts, tens of thousands of others will be the beneficiaries.

There are two of this breed whom I wish to particularly mention. To Mike Barrett, news reporter and editor, who resides in Burlington, Washington: Thank you, Mike. And David Call. Dave is a former attorney, accountant, and friend who burned the midnight oil until his face turned white and black shiners appeared under his eyes in reflection of his intense effort to ready this manuscript, while still keeping his dignity and good humor. In the wee hours of the last early morning: Thank you, Dave.

Foreword

Do you see the challenges in your life as stumbling blocks or stepping stones? We are all faced with challenges— whether they are physical, mental, or spiritual; or concern our relationships, work, finances, etc. We can let them get the best of us or we can turn them into opportunities to learn, grow, and share. I know of no other challenge that shakes us to the depth of our soul more than to be given the diagnosis of a terminal physical condition.

Tom Warren turned an incredible challenge into a journey of learning. He followed his heart when he knew there was more that could be done than what the doctors had told him. He studied and pushed himself to gain knowledge and insight into ways he could unravel the complex environmental prison he found himself trapped in. Now he is sharing with all of us what he can, to help us if we are searching for ways to improve our health.

I have been a dentist for over twelve years. During the last six years, I have not placed a silver-mercury filling into any tooth. The reason is simple: mercury is a poison that should not be used in a person's mouth. The scientific research overwhelmingly supports my stand. However, the American Dental Association believes that not *enough* mercury comes out of fillings to be a problem. I have a Mercury Vapor Analyzer that accurately measures the mercury-vapor release from fillings in the mouth. Daily, I get readings that are above the Occupational Safety and Health Administration's standards for an occupational-setting exposure. This means that many people are walking around breathing mercury vapors at levels that would shut down industries.

I have helped many people reduce their exposure to environmental stress. The best results come when a person is willing to himself take on the responsibility for his own health and to use me and other supportive health practitioners as helpers along his journey.

I would like to share just a couple of the rewarding experiences I have had recently.

A man whom I will call "John" had been searching for better health for about two years. He quit smoking cigarettes and drinking alcohol, and he saw a naturopathic doctor who helped him fight a problem with Candida and food allergies. His health improved, but he still was plagued by the following symptoms: overweight; "spacy feelings" and a very poor memory, especially short-term; mental confusion, with difficulty concentrating; teeth clenching; and headaches. In addition, his girlfriend and fellow workers were very irritated by his quick temper and lack of patience. He didn't seem to be able to handle stress at all. With a proper diet, vitamin and mineral supplementation, and the sequential replacement of his fillings, John noticed relief from his headaches, an improved memory, more energy, and the ability to control his appetite. Most of all, his girlfriend found him much nicer to have around since he no longer had such a quick temper and she didn't need to repeat herself all of the time. Also, John's fellow workers reported an increase in his energy and a new ability to remain levelheaded. John has added that he felt "the fog had lifted."

Another case concerns a woman whom I will call "Jane." She had what doctors told her was arthritis of the spine and lived with daily back pain for many years. I recommended she see a naturopath, and she was treated for a problem with Candida. The back pain left and has not returned. Jane also had been trying to conceive for over six years without success. She and her husband had been working with a specialist and tried everything short of *in vitro fertilization*. I recommended they read the book *Infertility and Birth Defects: Is Mercury From Silver Dental Fillings an Unsuspected Cause?* by Sam Ziff and Michael F. Ziff, D.D.S. The couple had their silver-mercury fillings replaced, and Jane became pregnant.

I commend Tom Warren for his fantastic job of bringing together all of the pieces of information that he has. We are all given challenges in life. My hope is that you, too, will see them as opportunities to learn and become your best. This book can help all of you reach for the resources and knowledge to support your journey and search for better health and a happier life.

Russ Borneman, D.D.S.
Anacortes, Washington

Preface

Getting well again is not easy. There are no short cuts. If the reader is unwilling or unable to make a real effort to change his lifestyle, nothing I have written will help him. This book may be a waste of money.

I cannot guarantee that what is contained in this book will "cure" you. However, I know it cured me, and I have seen others improve dramatically using this approach. Other Alzheimer's patients, and patients with schizophrenia, epilepsy, arthritis, and multiple sclerosis, have improved dramatically using the information contained herein, and I have had the pleasure of watching them move on with their lives.

I have letters from Alzheimer's victims who are happy to be breathing and celebrating life again. One woman with short-term-memory loss was ninety-nine years old. In her daughter's words, "Mother became absolutely lucid and clearly aware."

A gentleman, whom I'll call "Jim," was extensively tested and diagnosed by four different neurologists as having Alzheimer's. His family physician of twenty-five years concurred. His wife wrote, "I had arranged to put [Jim] in a nursing home as I could no longer deal with him. . . . I am most delighted to say, I canceled the reservation. You literally saved [Jim's] life. Thank you."

In 1984, schizophrenia was reversed in a patient who had been unresponsive to every conventional treatment conceivable for six years—within *four hours*. In another case, a friend of mine was in a state mental hospital for thirty-five years. His psychiatrists followed most of my instructions, and the gentleman recovered in less than *three months*.

I met a lovely woman, Janet Rule, who is now recovered from multiple sclerosis. She had been bedridden and unable to feed herself, wash herself, or use a bedpan without assistance. She even died and was resuscitated. Several months later, however, she recovered so quickly that she was able to drive her own car, by herself, within forty-eight hours after treatment. "I was driving down the street, doing everything I normally do," she said.

Another woman was sitting by a table, her head upon its surface. Slobber drained from her mouth. She tried to turn to greet me but could only raise her head three or four inches. Her feet were turned under like those of a mortally wounded bird. Her physician had canceled half of her appointments for two weeks in her efforts to save the patient, but she told me she was losing the patient by the hour. The young woman, however, did recover—starting just *two hours* after oral surgeons removed the metal from her mouth, gums, and jawbone. She is leading a normal life today.

There are many similar stories. Too many. . . .

I urge people with the diseases discussed here to seek advice and treatment from a medical doctor of their choosing—and to bring this book to that doctor's attention.

Beating Alzheimer's is primarily directed to Alzheimer's and schizophrenia patients and to those who love and care for them. However, there are many other medical complications that mimic Alzheimer's or schizophrenia, or cause additional mental problems that are reversible. For example, atherosclerosis can be reversed by chelation therapy, time-release niacin, and diet changes. The traditional American medical community is not familiar with chelation therapy, which removes metal from the brain and atherosclerosis from the arteries, but in some parts of Europe, heart-bypass surgery is not permitted until the patient has had at least twenty chelation treatments.

Daniel Hall, M.D., medical director of the American Association of Retired Persons (AARP), concurs. Dr. Hall says that long-standing disorders of the endocrine glands—particularly of the lungs, kidneys, and liver—including diabetes, may affect the brain. When these diseases are treated and controlled, he says, the dementia symptoms may end.

I hope that professionals will be able to use the information presented in this book. I hope and expect that they will be able to improve the medical treatments currently available to Alzheimer's and other patients. And I hope that the insights they gain will confirm the accuracy and quality of my presentation.

Introduction

Alzheimer's is murder. It mentally cripples millions each year. It devastates the patient and the family. It "arrives" out of nowhere, with no real warning, no explanation, and no hope for recovery. At least, this has been the thinking in traditional medical circles—until now.

Not that we are not working on it. We are. There is a national campaign to eradicate Alzheimer's disease. But to effect a cure for anything, we must first have a clear idea of *what* it is. Miss that initial step—identifying the *what*— and the *hows* and *whys* and *cures* never quite fall into place.

Many of the discoveries and inventions of the twentieth century have come about because someone was able to call upon knowledge from more than one field of study in a way no one had been able to do before and use that multidisciplinary approach to put together the pieces of a puzzle that was previously thought unsolvable. It is one of the disadvantages of progress that we become so specialized in one field, we have blinders on for the truths of any other field.

I believe the solution to Alzheimer's has eluded the medical profession and the best research laboratories not because of a lack of effort or sincerity, but because the answer lies in a multidisciplinary approach.

My opinions, naturally, differ from those of traditional medical practitioners. Do not expect most traditional medical specialists—for example, psychiatrists, neurologists, and dentists—to understand or support my presentation. Physicians even disagree among themselves on the proper approach to the treatment of chronic disease, depending on their individual education, training, and exposure to different medical specialties. Most traditional physicians and Alzheimer's researchers either tell me that Alzheimer's is incurable or seem to be stuck within the view of their particular medical specialty and have a difficult time seeing beyond it.

What is needed is to step back and look at the picture through a larger window. The answer does not lie within the scope of any one profession but rather in a unique combination of several.

In my view, unless there is *definite* medical evidence uncovered during a complete neurological and medical examination, neurology—as preposterous as it may seem—is not the correct medical specialty to treat Alzheimer's disease.

When the methods that traditional physicians are currently using fail to bring relief *and the doctor cannot detect the root cause of the problem,* many of the patient's complaints are often labeled as neurotic. This is precisely the clue that indicates the patient needs to see a new kind of doctor, such as a clinical ecologist (environmental allergist), orthomolecular psychiatrist or physician, or dental detoxicologist, *particularly* if Alzheimer's disease is suspected.

Most medical specialties are interdependent. By themselves, they cannot completely reverse a disease process.

Ten years ago, members of the Washington State Legislature, responsible for funding our state-run mental hospitals, told me there had been no breakthroughs in the treatment of mental disease in more than twenty-five years. They were very pessimistic.

Dr. Abram Hoffer, the internationally famous orthomolecular psychiatrist from Victoria, British Columbia, Canada, who wrote *Nutrients to Age Without Senility,* told me, "If you have only five minutes of lucid thought process, Alzheimer's is reversible." I have found that he is correct, and the information presented herein is both a critical breakthrough and a key that can help medical professionals begin to unlock not only the mysteries of Alzheimer's and schizophrenia, but many chronic diseases.

You will be surprised at how many other ailments vanish by using the same methods that reversed Alzheimer's disease in me. For example, my arthritis has reversed itself to a point where I am surprised when I do feel a little stiff once in a while. Painful hemorrhoids that plagued me for nearly thirty years and adult-onset diabetes have also both disappeared. My blood pressure has dropped from 147/90 to 117/70; my pulse has slowed from 100 to 70. The heart irregularities that I had since childhood vanished in an instant during the removal of an amalgam fragment from my jawbone.

Please understand that there is a point beyond which disease cannot be reversed. Afflicted patients usually do not approach alternative-practice physicians until they have exhausted all hope of recovery through traditional medicine, and a certain percentage of them do die. This is particularly true regarding cancer.

A doctor explained it to me this way: If the patient has had chemotherapy, the prognosis is unfavorable. A lot of money is involved in the traditional treatment of cancer, and alternative-practice specialists are reluctant to take on as a new patient someone who has exhausted all hope of recovery. Invariably, some of these patients have diseases that are too advanced to be treated successfully. The American Medical Association (AMA), American Dental Association (ADA), cancer and medical societies, attorneys, and surviving relatives are usually more than an alternative-practice physician cares to contend with.

So, I am not guaranteeing that even if you follow the regimen outlined in this book to the letter, you (or your loved one) will recover. But I did, and others have. Considering the bleak prognosis for Alzheimer's disease, anything is worth a try, isn't it? Especially if it has proven successful with others.

Do you (or does your loved one) have five minutes of lucid thought process? In other words, can the afflicted person carry on a reasonably normal conversation for five minutes? If so, go for it!

Earlier, I mentioned that the first task in solving a problem or curing a disease is to get a handle on *what* it is. By reviewing the events and symptoms that preceded my Alzheimer's, we'll explore *what* Alzheimer's is. Then we'll examine *how* it comes about, and *why* the teeth, diet, and family tree are such important parts of the diagnosis and treatment. While we are covering these topics, you will also be gathering the information necessary to start taking your (or your loved one's) situation in hand and to get appropriate treatment to start down the road to recovery.

I do want to make it clear before we start that this book is meant to serve as merely an introduction to this whole area. By the time you finish reading it, you should have a basic understanding. To make this approach really work, you will have to do, to a certain extent, what I did: you will need to read and study further. At the very minimum, you should acquire at least the first six of the following extraordinarily important books for Alzheimer's sufferers, which I call "must-read books." Read them all several times, then keep them handy for reference. The last five books, as you can see, are optional, but I strongly recommend them.

On dental detoxicology
- *It's All in Your Head*, by Hal A. Huggins, D.D.S. and Sharon A. Huggins

On clinical ecology
- *An Alternative Approach to Allergies*, by Theron G. Randolph, M.D., and Ralph W. Moss, Ph.D.
- *The Yeast Connection: A Medical Breakthrough*, by William G. Crook, M.D.

On orthomolecular medicine
- *Nutrition and Vitamin Therapy*, by Michael Lesser, M.D.
- *Nutrients to Age Without Senility*, by Abram Hoffer, M.D., Ph.D., and Morton Walker, D.P.M.
- *Feed Yourself Right*, by Lendon Smith, M.D.
- *Mega-Nutrition: The New Prescription for Maximum Health, Energy and Longevity*, by Richard A. Kunin, M.D.

Optional
- *Dr. Mandell's 5-Day Allergy Relief System*, by Marshall Mandell, M.D., and Lynne Waller Scanlon (on clinical ecology)

- *Why Do I Feel So Awful?* by David R. Collison, M.D. (on clinical ecology)
- *Dr. Mandell's Lifetime Arthritis Relief System*, by Marshall Mandell, M.D. (on clinical ecology)
- *Your Body Doesn't Lie*, by John Diamond, M.D. (to help you save money)
- *The McDougall Plan*, by John A. McDougall, M.D., and Mary A. McDougall (on nutrition and disease, especially cancer)

As we go along, I'll introduce you to the must-read books. Their authors are all pre-eminent professionals in their respective fields, and I have had the opportunity to personally seek out several of them for treatment. You, too, will come to know the importance of their work.

1.

The Elusive Thing
Called Alzheimer's

*There is something we do not understand about
mental illness. We think people are a lot more
responsible for their actions than they actually
are.*

—Father Allen Amirault
Psychologist, professor, friend

I do not remember much about that time. The memories
are there but I cannot deal with the pain of thinking of
them, so I push them off into a little corner beyond conscious thought and just go on. But if remembering will
help just one person, I will be happy to try.

THE DIAGNOSIS

On the morning of June 11, 1983, my family doctor sent
me to St. Peter Hospital, in Olympia, Washington, for a
computer assisted tomograph (CAT) scan. Three little
girls, with their mother and grandmother, played in the

waiting room, talking, giggling, so infectiously full of life. When my examination was finished, I asked the nurse if she would mind if I waited for the attending doctor to read the x-rays and tell me the results. She made a gallant effort to remain serene, but her face had a desolation I had seen before: on my wife Louise's face the day we lost our daughter Lisa. After a long moment, the nurse told me my family doctor would relay the results to me. But from the look on her face, I knew them already: I had Alzheimer's disease.

The Alzheimer's report and x-rays (see Figures 1.1 and 1.2, on pages 10 and 11) are so innocuous that no one but a physician might realize they are actually the diagnosis of Alzheimer's disease, the prognosis of which is as final as any death warrant ever written. Until now, there has never been a reprieve.

The following Monday, my family physician, Dr. Endre Mihalyi, quietly explained what was happening to my brain. Trying to be as objective and hopeful as possible, he said that I "might have as long as seven years to live." I appreciated his kindness and thoughtful consideration in what was obviously a painful prognosis for both of us.

A few days later, I had my x-rays read by another physician at St. Peter. He pointed to the brain atrophy the CAT scan had revealed and said there was no doubt about the accuracy of the report.

The next evening, I watched a nationally televised documentary about Alzheimer's disease. While I cannot tell you much about the program, Louise says it made me terribly depressed.

Neither do I remember when, or even where, I saw the picture. Maybe in a book. It was a photograph of a long-haired black cat in a glass box about three and a half feet wide and two feet high. The animal was backed so tightly into a corner that its tail and body were squished up against the ceiling of the cage. Only its two front paws touched the floor. Its hair, from its head to its tail and across its shoulders, was standing straight up. Its mouth was slobbering, and its eyes were fixed—as if formed from glass—on a little white mouse sitting in the middle of the cage. At the bottom of the photograph was written something about an LSD experiment.

Whenever I try to remember my reaction to my diagnosis, the photograph, or the Alzheimer's television program, the only impressions I have are of the pain of knowing, of the cat's fear, and of the sorrow over the devastation my Alzheimer's disease would cause my family.

So, forgive me for not remembering more about that time.

I have looked into the face of death many times and walked away, but death usually brushes on by in an instant and is nearly as quickly forgotten. I remember being sad only once, not at the prospect of dying, but for the need to make a positive contribution.

What I do remember is that I felt like I had been beaten up by Joe Louis. Progressively, my thinking process evaporated. I was so exhausted, there were times that I had to crawl up the stairs. My head ached. Occasionally, my brain felt like it was burning. My handwriting deteriorated. I became a cantankerous grouch. I experienced a rapidly diminishing capacity to remember names and usually had to look up my own phone number; sometimes I became too confused to complete the task. Conversation was really difficult, especially for the unlucky person I was talking with because I constantly asked questions that had been answered just minutes before and then forgot what the subject was about.

I prayed to die but after a while began to realize that I would have to go through it all, including the end stages of

ST. PETER HOSPITAL
OLYMPIA, WASHINGTON

MR # _____   X-RAY # 5066-83   Pt # 3-47004-7

Name WARREN, Tom   Age 50   Room No Rad.   Date of Study 6/11/83

Radiograph of   CT head scan

Other Information   R/O atrophy/Alzheimers   Ref Phys   Mihalyl

CT HEAD SCAN

Noncontrast and contrast enhanced scans were obtained No high or low
density lesions are identified No abnormal mass effect Ventricles are
normal in size and configuration Mild frontal and temporal lobe atrophy is
noted with widened sylvian and interhemispheric fissures Normal posterior
fossa

IMPRESSION Very mild bilateral frontal and temporal lobe atrophy No other
abnormalities seen

DRJ cac
6/12/83
_____
                        D R James, M D

768-83-S-4

X-RAY REPORT

Figure 1.1.   First x-ray report, with diagnosis of Alzheimer's
disease.

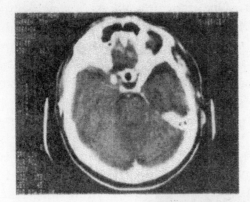

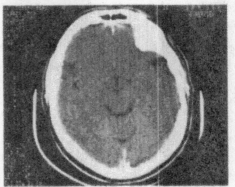

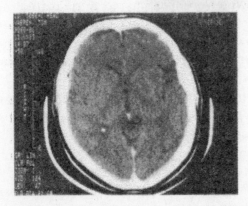

Figure 1.2. First x-rays, which show brain atrophy and Alzheimer's.

the disease process. One morning when I was feeling particularly miserable, I asked the Lord that if I had to die this death, to help me be the means through which the cure for Alzheimer's disease would be found. And in his infinite grace and mercy, God answered both of my prayers.

I sought out a variety of medical specialists. I read voraciously on the subject, devouring books, pamphlets, and research papers, most of which I immediately forgot. But even though my brain was barely functioning and I would forget almost everything I read within thirty seconds, somehow I picked up a tidbit here and a scrap there. And when I felt an intuitive nudge or recognized a whisper of hope, I marked the book, and talked it over with Louise when she came home from her job at the pharmacy.

The most important thing I learned was to accept the responsibility for my own health—to read, study, and think for myself. Every person I have met who has recovered from a chronic disease has had this same attitude.

Finally, a pattern began to emerge, even to my befogged brain. So I began to ask questions—more specific questions—of those who were treating me, and I tested the theories I was reading about on myself. I became my own guinea pig. Somehow, with a lot of help from Louise and various allergy groups, I began to take charge of my own recovery.

As I've said, I am not a medical professional, just an ordinary man who wanted desperately to live a useful life. And just as in the case of most anything new, "the establishment" didn't believe there was a cure and wouldn't encourage my efforts. We—my wife, the allergy groups, and the few doctors and other professionals who were espousing the treatment regimen I was discovering—were considered to be practicing voodoo. The professionals involved were, at the time, thought of as mavericks in traditional medical circles. Thank God for this new breed of hero!

Not that I blame the medical profession. Doctors must put their trust in their traditional training and in the research capabilities of the gigantic pharmaceutical laboratories. They cannot accept every story that comes down the pike. They must wait to see them confirmed.

Well, I couldn't wait. My condition could become irreversible while I waited for someone else to develop the cure for me.

It is my sincere hope that medical professionals will read this book—and take notice of it—now. My toil has paid off. After getting an idea of what my treatment maybe should be, I asked one of my physicians to perform the Heidelberg Stomach Acid Test,[1] which indicated that my stomach acid was more neutral than water. The physician shook his head in amazement; he had been giving up more and more hope for my recovery as my memory processes became worse. The test was the first indication that my Alzheimer's could be reversed; it was the first step on my road to recovery. You see, it was the first hint that what was wrong with me had a metabolic base: neutral stomach acid does not break down food correctly. No matter how good a quality of food I was eating, since my stomach acid was neutral, the food wasn't being digested properly and the nutrients weren't getting to my brain and body. To put it bluntly, my brain was starving to death.

Nearly four years later—years of agony, frustration, and depression, but also of hard work, hope, and improvement—on April 4, 1987, a new CAT scan indicated the disease process had reversed. (See Figures 1.3 and 1.4, on pages 14 and 15.) I had the test results checked by several specialists. So shocked was one physician that his hand

ST. PETER HOSPITAL
OLYMPIA, WASHINGTON

MR # ____81375____   Image # __5066__   Pt # ___7-42392-1___

Name _WARREN, Tom_ Age _54_ Room No _RAD_ Date of Study _4/30/87_

Study of ___HeadCT_____

Other Information ____Alzheimers____ Ref Phys __/BUSHER/KIRKLAND__

CT OF THE HEAD without contrast shows normal sized unshifted ventricles
Cavum septum No atrophy appreciated

IMPRESSION   Negative CT

WJM:jjc 4/30/87 1700   W.J. MIKKELSEN, MD

768-83-S-5

IMAGING REPORT

Figure 1.3.   Second x-ray report, with diagnosis of no brain
atrophy and negative findings.

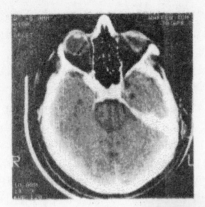

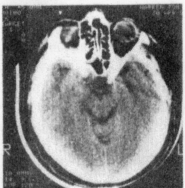

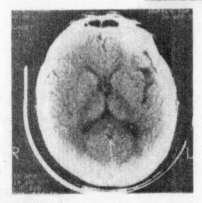

Figure 1.4. Second x-rays, which show that the Alzheimer's had reversed.

shook as he pointed to the new x-ray plates. I asked him whether he had ever heard of recovery before. He answered with a simple "no."

Another doctor, a neurologist, refused to believe that I had ever had the disease because I was not dead. A neuropathologist said I had never had Alzheimer's but that I did have, and still have, mild brain atrophy. He said that x-rays are not considered definitive by themselves.

I have had my x-rays checked by several radiologists, all of whom said there was definite shrinkage and lesions that are not now present but who refused to confirm their observations. One of them said, "You're just stuck."

I do not have the slightest doubt in my mind that I actually did have Alzheimer's disease. Nor do I have a question that I came very close to an irreversible prognosis. I am living proof that death is *not* the only alternative. In me, the disease was reversed. I enjoy the fruits of active, joy-filled days again. I once more appreciate sunsets, remember names, drive a car, converse with friends, think, and plan. More importantly, however, I have returned to work after an absence of eleven years.

AN ALLERGIC RESPONSE

The average person sees Alzheimer's as personality change, memory loss, and senility. But these are the apparent results—the symptoms—not the disease. What is Alzheimer's, the Disease? What causes it? When does it start? Is it hereditary?

Alzheimer's disease is characterized by tangled nerve fibers and plaque in the brain.[2] Plaque is residue that leaches through swollen membranes and hardens as the swelling reaction diminishes. Researchers of Alzheimer's disease have found broken nerve endings encased in plaque residue, which seems consistent with the leaching process during a swelling reaction. But what causes the swelling?

In 1986, Senetek PLC, a California-based biotechnology firm, announced that it had developed the first known test for Alzheimer's.[3] The test measures an antigen found in the cerebrospinal fluid bathing the brain. Cerebrospinal fluid is the serumlike fluid that flows through the connected cavities and canals of the brain and spinal cord. Antigens are any substance—a food, pollen, or dust, for example—that during an allergic reaction, stimulates the production of antibodies or reacts with them. Swelling is often a symptom of an allergic reaction.

Chemical sensitivities are different from allergic reactions in that the body is unable to produce antibodies against the chemicals or metals to which it is sensitive. The patient, though, suffers similar distress. For practical purposes, I will refer to both actual allergic reactions and chemical sensitivities as "allergic reactions." I will refer to metal poisoning using the metal's specific name, e.g., mercury toxicity or lead toxicity.

Research findings connecting Alzheimer's to allergies are continuing to come in. In 1987, Dr. James Gusella, a researcher, announced the discovery of an Alzheimer's genetic marker. A defective gene was found in approximately 10 percent of Alzheimer's patients. However, Dr. Gusella also indicated that in many cases, the gene may not cause Alzheimer's but might instead act in concert with some other factor, possibly environmental, "such as aluminum or some other environmental factor."[4]

In September 1988, researchers at the University of British Columbia, in Victoria, British Columbia, Canada, reported discovering that some parts of the brain in Alzheimer's patients are more heavily afflicted than other parts and that a large amount of a certain element is found in the heavily afflicted parts. The element, microglia, is

classically found where the body is attempting to fight off
a foreign substance. The researchers concluded that the
activity they discovered indicated "an active chronic inflammatory process" in Alzheimer's disease. What does
that mean? We all recognize the word "active." "Chronic"
means "continuing," "ongoing." "Inflammatory" refers to
swelling.

Then in February 1991, the British science magazine
Nature reported that researchers at Saint Mary's Hospital
Medical School, in London, have identified a genetic mu-
tation that affects the body's production of an amyloid
protein. They do not know the cause of the genetic muta-
tion, but I believe they will eventually prove that it is
metal and chemical toxicity.

Swelling in the brain is an allergic reaction to an antigen. It takes place at the nerve endings within the brain.
The nerve endings, called "synapses," are where the
nerve impulses pass between the nerves. As the immediate area swells, thought transmission becomes garbled,
causing bizarre behavior and hallucinations.[5] This swelling had been noticed during brain operations, but until
recently, no one knew what the phenomenon indicated.

Dr. Bernard S. Zussman, of Memphis, Tennessee, reports the story of an allergic patient with an opening in his
skull from an operation. Whenever the patient ate something to which he was allergic, his brain would swell,
expanding out through the surgical hole and pushing up
the overlying scalp. This was an immeasurably important
observation.[6]

The July 2, 1990, issue of *U.S. News and World Report,* in an article by Shannon Browniee entitled "The
Body at War: Baring the Secrets of the Immune System,"
says, "More lethal still is the poisonous surfeit of hormones
produced by the overreacting immune system. These hormones, called lymphokines, make mischief in surrounding

tissue and organs, causing swelling and fever. . . . The effect of superantigens is so murderously swift. . . ."

Headaches are a common symptom of cerebral (brain-related) allergies. I asked a man who had been hospitalized for schizophrenia for more than twenty years what he does to relieve his headaches. He takes Dristan, a decongestant/antihistamine-combination that reduces swelling and has an analgesic to combat pain.

Clinical ecologists have been successfully treating schizophrenia—which they call cerebral allergies, brain fog (spaciness), brain fag (fatigue), or brain allergies—for more than thirty years. At least 60 percent of cerebral-allergy patients are said to recover when correctly diagnosed and tested. Another 10 percent partially recover, allowing a reasonable degree of clear thinking and successful living very far into the disease process.

Dr. Theron Randolph, the prominent clinical ecologist from Chicago (now retired), specialized in treating patients with a multitude of chronic diseases whom other physicians had given up on. His average patient had been treated by fifty different health professionals before arriving at his hospital unit. Dr. Randolph found, after treating more than 20,000 patients in his unit, that less than 20 percent of those admitted with complaints of mental disorders needed continued psychotherapy.

What does all this point to? What have we learned? Let's review.

- The major symptoms of Alzheimer's are caused by tangled nerve fibers and plaque in the brain.
- Microglia, antigens, and swelling are physical responses to something to which the body is allergic.
- Noted scientists, though searching for a genetic cause, recognize that an environmental (i.e., allergic) factor is involved.

- When schizophrenia, Alzheimer's, and neurological problems have been approached as allergy-related, great—even tremendous—progress has been made.

What reasonable conclusion can you reach when faced with these facts?

Dr. Mohammed Nasser, a specialist in preventive medicine, internal medicine, and cardiology at the Nasser Medical Center, in Lake Villa, Illinois, put it in a nutshell when he said, "Alzheimer's is an autoimmune response."[7]

This points to a real cure for Alzheimer's disease and schizophrenia, and other brain-related "diseases" as well. We should concentrate our attention on cerebral-allergy sources (and perhaps even change the names of these conditions to "advanced cerebral allergies") and dispense appropriate treatments.

ALZHEIMER'S IN MY LIFE

Finally understanding that Alzheimer's is connected with allergies surely explained a lot of things I had never before understood about my family and myself.

My Family History

As Dr. Gusella pointed out, Alzheimer's disease does not always have a genetic base (cause). In fact, in only 10 percent of Alzheimer's patients is a defective gene labeled as "the cause." Gusella suspects that in a higher percentage of victims, a weak gene is interacting with, or affected by, environmental factors, i.e., more people have allergic reactions.

What about that 10 percent of patients whose Alzheimer's is said to be "caused" by the defective gene? You will learn, as we proceed, that some of the foreign substances, particularly metals, that enter the brain, and which the body attempts to stave off, head directly for the weakest gene and work to destroy it. When that task is accomplished, the patient is not only sensitized (super-susceptible) to all kinds of foreign substances and allergic reactions, but he also passes the susceptibility down to his progeny through the defective gene.[8] The defective gene is probably the cause of the susceptibility to allergies, but the allergies, and the body's response to them, are what bring on the symptoms of Alzheimer's.

It is clinically accepted, and studies have proven, that many diseases tend to cluster within family groups.[9] This is generally referred to as the hereditary nature of an illness. As you might expect, my family has a long history of cerebral-allergic response.

My grandmother was a dear, senile old woman. But then, in her time, senility was thought to be an unavoidable part of growing old. Her daughter, my mother, exhibited schizophrenic behavior from my earliest memory. Mother would sit up all night, her feet resting on the door of an old-fashioned wood-and-coal stove and her body wrapped tightly in sleeping bags. She would surround herself with an elaborate wall of furniture, including, behind the leather chair in which she slept, a heavy, five-foot-high, early-model radio. To complete the enclosure, she would place chicken wire over everything. She would leave the windows wide open and wrap chiffon scarves around her head and face because, she claimed, people were gassing her at night.[10] During the day, Mother would carry her food around in laundry bags, which she watched constantly, afraid someone was trying to poison her. She would always turn on the tap full-force for three or four minutes before taking a drink in order, she would say, to get the "dope" out of the water.

Psychiatrists often tell schizophrenic patients that they have no insight into their emotional problems. Mother's behavior proved she actually had more insight into her psychosis than any of her physicians or family members ever gave her credit for.[11]

We constantly badgered Mother, telling her that she could get better if she would "only try." Our lack of understanding, however, caused her great distress.[12] We did not realize she was already doing the best she could. We thought Mother had control over her behavior because, at the time, we could not recognize what is now apparent: there was an allergenic/environmental/nutritional connection that put her actions beyond our understanding.

My mother's brother also had problems. My uncle, who passed away twenty years ago, was a fine old man who took care of my mother, two sisters, and me after my father deserted us during the Depression. Uncle Bill was an electrician who enjoyed solving complicated mathematical equations late at night. During and after World War II, he worked very hard in the shipyards around Puget Sound in Washington State. He was exceptionally well liked, but those who worked with him recognized that his thinking process moved in slow motion.[13] His foremen usually assigned him the menial task of setting up the lights by which the other electricians would see. Uncle Bill constantly complained of breathing difficulties because the welding fumes choked him, and he tried to stay away from welding as much as possible. He finally suffered a mental breakdown from overwork and lack of sleep while attempting to save the family business after Grandfather died unexpectedly. Mother said he was never quite the same afterward.

My younger sister committed suicide at age forty-five. She seemed very angry, the same way I was at the onset of my Alzheimer's. It would be easy to assume that a defective gene is the root cause of my family's mental complaints. In addition to a possible defective gene, all of these medical problems might also be linked to iatrogenic disease.

My Personal Story

This is not a story where everybody lives happily ever after, as in a children's fable. It does not work that way with schizophrenia or Alzheimer's disease.

A notion exists in medical circles that Alzheimer's disease suddenly strikes a person during midlife. That may be the time when Alzheimer's disease is recognized, but in my experience, vague symptoms begin as early as age eight. In my case, in the third grade, I stammered so badly that I was unable to utter more than thirty words in school all year. Speech therapy compounded the problem rather than helping it.

In the sixth grade, my formerly precise handwriting became scribbled and scratchy.[14] Writing, by the way, is a cerebral-motor function. At the time, no one realized there was a connection between handwriting, dyslexia, stuttering, and cerebral diseases such as Alzheimer's.

At age six, I had suffered a severe head injury in an automobile accident, which was suspected to be the possible cause of my stuttering. I was finally hospitalized in the eighth grade so an electroencephalogram (EEG) could be run on me. The EEG revealed no abnormalities, but head injuries are suspected to be a part of the pathology of Alzheimer's disease.

In the ninth grade, I began falling asleep in class. I thought my teachers were dull. My attitude and grades plummeted. I stammered. Skin dissolved in large areas on my face. The skin on my arms became blotchy and itchy. I scratched, causing many scabs to form.[15] I began skipping school.

Early in 1961, I experienced a severe mental break-down and became involved with the law (robbery) be-cause of overwork, exhaustion, lack of sleep, a failing marriage, a lousy value system, and most important, the stimulant known as "speed," which was administered under medical supervision to help me stay awake in order to continue working long hours. I was found not guilty, but was declared mentally ill and committed to Eastern State Hospital, at Medical Lake, Washington.

Many years later, after I straightened out my life and moved on with my education and career in the insurance industry, I walked out of an important accounting class because I could not stay awake. I thought the professor—who, incidentally, was considered to be among the finest in Washington—was so dull, he put me to sleep.[16] I found out later that it was necessary to discover the reasons behind all of these symptoms before I could move forward and begin to reverse my Alzheimer's.

My road to recovery has been like trying, while blind-folded, to find every one of two hundred sewing needles in a haystack. Every needle has been addictive, difficult, and painful to let go of. Moreover, because of my par-ticular exposure to foods, chemicals, and toxins, com-paratively few needles have caused the same symptoms in me as they would in someone else. No two people are identical in their symptoms.

Luckily, there is a general approach that does work to reverse the disease process within most individuals. I know, because it worked for me and I have seen it work, sometimes dramatically, for other people with symptoms similar to mine.

The books I read indicated that the many lifestyle changes required for recovery would become easier as time progressed. Within eighteen months, these pro-cedures became a part of my family's natural living pattern. My health, after several years, has so improved that I can say, in all honesty, that being able to feel good again has been worth all the pain and struggle. The road to recovery is not an easy path or a straight line, nor is it fast. Rather, it is a cobblestone road of many tiny lifestyle changes, each another step toward renewed vitality and clarity of thought.

Then one fine day, your neurologist will say that you never had Alzheimer's disease, as mine did. A neuropathologist told me why: neurologists regard Alzheimer's as any memory disease they cannot cure.

Never mind what diagnosis your physician blessed you with. Your mental health and memory can improve. Mine did.

2.

Your Own Teeth May Be Your Worst Enemy

Teeth and brain are close neighbors—at a distance of only a few inches.

—Dr. Patrick Störtebecker
Swedish neurologist and author

Approximately twelve years ago, a Colorado dentist made a bombshell rediscovery that many of the 20 percent of Dr. Theron Randolph's patients who did not respond to treatment may actually have had an iatrogenic disease. Dr. Hal Huggins discovered that silver fillings, which are actually amalgam compounds containing 52 percent mercury, a metal incredibly toxic to humans, leach mercury. How did Dr. Huggins' colleagues and the ADA react to his monumental discovery? The February 1988 issue of *Let's Live* magazine has an article by the late Carlton Fredericks, Ph.D., entitled "Organized Dentistry's Poisonality," which reads, in part:

Dentists concerned about the toxicity from silver amalgam fillings have been made outcasts by the

American Dental Association (ADA) exactly as they were nearly a century ago when organized dentistry literally outlawed those who were concerned about amalgam fillings.

The Swedish Social Welfare and Health Administration, on May 20, 1987, announced that "amalgam is an unsuitable and toxic dental filling material and shall be discontinued as soon as suitable replacement materials are produced. At first step, amalgam work in pregnant women will be stopped."

However, on July 15, 1988, Sam Ziff, the editor and publisher of *Bio-Probe* magazine, sent a letter to my dentist that said, in part:

It is our understanding that the Swedish Health Board has taken a position supporting the use of amalgam even in pregnant women. This is a complete contradiction to the Health Board's public policy statements of May 20, 1987, as reported in the *Sevenska Dagbladet* of that date. Furthermore, it totally disregards the recommendations of the Swedish Expert Commission who concluded that amalgam was toxic and unsuitable as a dental filling material and that its use in pregnant women should be stopped.

One can only speculate as to why the Health Board has now reversed their previous public position. The basic scientific facts precipitating the recommendations of the Expert Commission have not changed. In fact, since the public release of the Expert Commission findings, several world toxicology experts on mercury have concluded that the release of mercury from dental amalgams makes the predominant contribution to human exposure to inorganic mercury. It is apparent that a tremendous amount of pressure has been brought to bear on the Health Board to cause them to reverse their previous public position.

Today, many patients, dentists, physicians and scientists from Australia to Alaska have recognized the toxic disaster caused by mercury within dental amalgam fillings. The clinical experience has been the same everywhere. Also the oppression exerted by the powerful dental organizations against patients and anti-amalgam dentists has repeated from country to country.

In my opinion, the dental community does recognize the fact that it has placed a deadly poison—mercury—in the mouths of nearly the total population. How could it not? The United States Environmental Protection Agency (EPA) requires dentists to store mercury in liquid, in a sealed jar. When a filling with mercury is removed from a tooth, the EPA says it is toxic waste and must be disposed of as such.

Luckily, the Swedish Parliament eventually held a public hearing on the use of silver-amalgam fillings, in October 1988. And in November 1990, the Swedish government announced that the National Health Plan will pay one-half the cost of replacing the fillings.

Why all the furor over mercury in a book about mental disease? Because mercury turned out to be a major part of my problem, as it has for so many of the people I have met through my work to combat Alzheimer's disease. In this chapter, I will try to explain exactly what mercury is and why it is dangerous. I will also describe the symptoms of mercury toxicity and what to do if you believe you (or your loved one) are a victim.

MERCURY, FILLINGS, AND TOXICITY

Dr. Hal Huggins, the Colorado dentist who rediscovered that silver-amalgam fillings leach mercury, is now waging an all-out campaign against mercury. He has switched his practice from filling teeth to diagnosing and treating mercury toxicity in dental patients. He says that everyone has a weak link, but that everyone has a different weak link, which is why the mercury–mental-health connection was not made until recently. If your weak link happens to be neurological, he says, then—bingo!—your neurological system gets zapped.

According to *Introduction to Urine Analysis*, a report that can be obtained from Dr. Huggins:

Dr. Jaro Pleva, Ph.D., of Sweden, who is a corrosion scientist and expert on mercury toxicity[1] has measured the amount of mercury remaining in five-year-old silver amalgam fillings and found approximately 27 percent mercury. [Remember: new fillings contain approximately 52 percent mercury.]

Twenty-year-old fillings were found to contain less than 5 percent mercury. The scientific community agrees that our bodies cannot withstand doses of over 100 micrograms of mercury daily.[2] Radics et al. in their studies found 150 micrograms leaching off mercury fillings daily.

Where does the mercury go? Part of it comes off the surface of a filling in the form of vapor.[3] As we inhale, this vapor enters our lungs and can be absorbed into our bloodstream. As we eat, it is incorporated into our food, swallowed, digested and absorbed into our bloodstream with access to our entire body.

Mercury is a toxic substance in its liquid and vapor forms, but there is another form that is considered 100 times more toxic, especially to the nervous system, a chemical form called methyl mercury.[4] Thomas Ely, M.D. said, "Methyl mercury is one of the most potent and insidious poisons in existence."

In *It's All in Your Head,* the first book on our must-read list, Dr. Huggins says:

A drug called Colchicine is the standard comparison for chemicals that produce birth defects and chromosomal damage. It is the strongest drug known for producing genetic problems. Methyl Mercury is also 1,000 times more toxic to the body than Colchicine.

You would think that older fillings are less toxic, but clinical ecologists know that after prolonged exposure to any toxic substance, even minuscule amounts may produce a very strong reaction. As an example, during provocative testing on me in the hospital clinical ecology unit in 1982, two drops of diluted chlorine under my tongue caused me to have the intense physical reaction of becoming paralyzed while having a hallucination. In provocative testing, an allergic patient first fasts, then is "challenged" with the suspect food or chemical. My allergic reaction stopped approximately five minutes after I was given oxygen. (Interestingly, a report by Sam Ziff in the March 1988 *Bio-Probe* points toward a connection between chlorine and silver fillings, further implicating mercury as a major cause of my allergic reactions.)

Another time, I was attending a meeting of mercury-sensitive individuals when a woman who had recovered from multiple sclerosis became ill from sitting next to another person who had a mouth full of amalgam fillings. The other person's breath "fouled the air" for her. The woman moved, and her symptoms disappeared. In addition, a number of dentists have had to retire from the dental profession because they have become too sensitive to mercury vapor to walk into a dental office.

Researchers have announced they are studying the olfactory nerves of Alzheimer's patients to look for what goes wrong early in the Alzheimer's disease process. Patrick Störtebecker, a Swedish neurologist, wrote in the March 1989 *Swedish Journal of Biological Medicine:*

> Baader and Holstein in 1933, and later Stock in 1936, reported insidious chronic poisoning from much lower Hg [mercury] levels gives a sensitivity toward further mercury exposure. Traces of mercury could produce symptoms, especially if the metal [or methyl mercury] was inhaled through the nose, etc.[5]

The November 11, 1988, issue of *Dental and Health Facts News Letter,* published by the Foundation for Toxic Free Dentistry, reports that a group of researchers at the University of Kentucky found increased mercury in Alzheimer's brain tissue. The Störtebecker Foundation for Research, in Stockholm, Sweden, reports that the high concentrations of metallic mercury found postmortem in the brain originate mainly from the mercury in dental amalgam fillings. However, far more dangerous are similarly released mercurial fumes, which settle in the mucous membranes of the upper region of the nasal cavity and are then transported directly to the brain.

A silver filling is composed of five dissimilar metals: 50 percent pure elemental mercury,[6] 35 percent silver, 13 percent tin, 2 percent copper, and a trace amount of zinc. When these dissimilar metals combine with saliva, a battery effect occurs. Studies indicate than an electrical current accelerates the release of hazardous mercury vapor.

A research paper entitled *Dental "Silver" Tooth Fill-*

ings: A Source of Mercury Exposure Revealed by Whole-Body Image Scan and Tissue Exposure was written by Leszek J. Hahn et al. and published on August 28, 1989, by the Departments of Radiology and Medical Physiology, University of Calgary, Alberta, Canada. It ended all speculation about the stability and dangers of silver fillings by reporting what happened when radioactive mercury-silver fillings were placed in the teeth of adult sheep. Mercury appeared in high concentrations in the sheeps' kidneys, livers, jaw tissue, and gastrointestinal tracts. It was found in lower concentrations in their frontal cortices, occipital cortices, thalami, cerebrospinal fluid, pituitary glands, thyroids, and adrenals. It was found throughout their whole bodies—within twenty-nine days. The average silver filling remains in a human mouth approximately seven to nine years. The researchers added that in the sheep, "In the central nervous system, the brain frontal cortex and thalamus, concentrations of mercury were higher than either the blood or cerebrospinal fluid."

In 1936, two researchers named Furman and Murray said, "A variety of radical reactions can be expected in a system with mercury, iron, copper, oxygen and reducing substances like ascorbic acid." Earlier, in 1907, a professor of pharmacology at Greifswald named Schultz had said:

Thus mercury can, in the presence of chlorine[7] or oxygen and living cells or tissues, intensely enhance the normal turnover of these [free radicals] substances. The changes in these basic processes by mercury is the cause of both the substantial medical effects and the toxicity of mercury.

The last paper quoted was published at the beginning of the century. Now, near the end of the century, the research and papers are continuing—not only continuing, but picking up steam. And they will continue to pick up steam until the evidence is accepted as proof.

Next, we will look at the symptoms of mercury toxicity.

THE SYMPTOMS OF MERCURY TOXICITY

The Summer 1987 issue of *Mothering* magazine features an article by Bill Wolfe, D.D.S., and Penny Davis Wolfe, R.N. Entitled "Fillings, Mercury and You," it lists several common symptoms of mercury sensitivity:

> The most common symptoms of mercury toxicity are central nervous disorders—depression, chronic fatigue, dizziness, frequent urination, insomnia, irritability, headaches, as well as chronic recurrent skin problems, metallic taste and depressed immune system. . . . The greatest advantage of composites [plastic fillings] is that they provide no mercury or [occasionally very low] electrogalvanism.

Patrick Störtebecker, the Swedish neurologist, has also compiled a list of symptoms signalling mercury toxicity. In his book *Neurology for Barefoot Doctors in All Countries: Correct Diagnosis by Simple Methods,*[8] he says, "The whole picture [mercury poisoning] is very often misinterpreted, and mercury intoxicated persons are being looked upon as suffering from "imaginary illnesses."

A few of the mental symptoms he lists are:

> Lack of strength, force—to resolve doubts and uncertainties, or to resist obsessions, compulsions, or phobias, that one knows are irrational.
>
> There is a conspicuous loss of memory, especially to "close" events. . . . Lack of concentration, insomnia, moodiness, the unpredictable and rapid changeableness of mood, e.g., "rage,"

especially uttered as sudden outbursts of anger . . . self-effacement, depression, and suicidal thoughts.

Other signs, according to Störtebecker, are a stuffy nose, dry crusts within the nose [and a tendency, therefore, to pick the nose], rhinitis, plugged ears, "chest pain,"[9] hyperventilation, increased urinary output, a lesion of the pituitary gland, *diabetes insipidus,* the feeling that the head is covered by a globe of glass, and chilly and shivery feelings.

I had sometimes noticed the globe-of-glass sensation on the top of my head. However, being constantly chilly and shivery has only been bothersome since my fillings were removed. Before, I was never cold. If anything, I continually complained of being too warm. A woman once told me she also had this problem after her fillings were removed but not before.

Although I am not a physician, and do not purport to be one, I have had the opportunity to speak with so many people during the last few years through my work with Alzheimer's that I have been able to compile my own list of possible symptoms. Again, I am **not** a doctor. Please discuss any symptoms or suspicions you may have with your personal physician, dental detoxicologist, or other health-care specialist.

Through my discussions of symptoms with the people I have met, I have noticed that there seems to be a definite pattern of subclinical signs indicating the possibility of a mercury-toxicity–allergy connection. For example, I have noticed that a white pallor of the face or puffy bags under the eyes may signify a food or pollen allergy or a chemical sensitivity. These, in turn, may cause cerebral allergic brain-fog reactions and all sorts of behavior problems that mental-health professionals never seem quite able to understand. Later on in life, these untreated food, pollen, or chemical allergies may produce problems with arthritis.

Dark circles under the eyes, called "shiners," may indicate hydrocarbon (e.g., gas, oil, wood, coal, newsprint, candles) sensitivities. They might also just signify the need for more sleep, however. Excessive urination; a heavy, fatigued feeling; sugar problems, such as low blood sugar or diabetes; underweight; and overweight can also be signs pointing toward mercury toxicity. Most mercury-toxic victims also seem to be plagued by an immoderate fascination with sweets.

Other subclinical clues I've noticed include white spots on the fingernails (zinc or calcium deficiency) and hang-nails (folic-acid deficiency). Ridges on the nails may denote a mineral deficiency. If you cannot remember your dreams, you may have a pyridoxine (vitamin B-6) deficiency. In this case, look at your tongue: a white growth there might suggest a Candida yeast infection. Your tongue should be smooth. Cracks, splits, or holes in your tongue signify an acute niacin (vitamin B-3) deficiency, a possible pyridoxine deficiency, or malabsorption of nutrients in general. Your fillings may be dark and corroded, or you may have a significant amount of other dental work. Sometimes, in very sick people, there may be mercury in the gums. Disfiguring acne scars also might be an indication of mercury irritation.

Scabs, or scars from scabs, on the arms may indicate mercury toxicity. Small white pustules on the forearms or back of the neck, or pustules or a red rash on the groin could indicate a Candida infection. Stomach distress—burning sensations, sharp pains, heartburn, flatulence—can also be an indication.

All of the subclinical signs I've mentioned could signify faulty digestion, food allergies, a depressed immune response, and mercury toxicity. If your fillings are dark and corroded, I would suggest taking the Heidelberg Stomach Acid Test and seeing a dental detoxicologist, clinical ecologist, or orthomolecular psychiatrist or physician. Even if all your teeth have already been pulled—and were pulled years ago—if you evidence at least some of the aforementioned symptoms, you should consider getting a panorex (dental x-ray) to find any amalgam fragments lodged in your gums or jawbone. Most dentists do not consider amalgam fragments important enough to bother with. They are!

In the beginning of my Alzheimer's treatment, I was unable to think clearly enough to cooperate in the healing process. Luckily, I found a homeopathic physician who helped me clear my thinking, restore my strength, and reverse my cantankerous disposition over a period of several months. I continued to improve for a year, until I moved with my family into a new apartment six years ago. Within a short time, my thought process and energy levels deteriorated until they were worse than before my first appointment with the physician. The doctor was shocked at my appearance on my next visit.

The only thing *I* noticed was different with my body, however, was that every time I ate, my stomach rumbled.

A woman I met in the hospital was allergic to *everything* in the environment. All of the patients and physicians expected her to die. We stayed in touch. Eventually, an internal specialist found that she did not have stomach acid to digest her food. It took a while, but she fully recovered. (One good result of our stay in the hospital clinical ecology unit is that we both learned a great deal about how to protect ourselves from environmental pollutants, chemicals, pollens, and foods.)

I decided to have my own stomach acid checked, and, if the Heidelberg Stomach Acid Test revealed nothing, to give up and die. As I suspected, my stomach acid proved

to be more neutral than water, and I recognized it was time
to try a different approach. I have also learned since then
that the latex paint in my family's new apartment was
contaminated with mercury. Mercury in latex paint out-
gasses continually, and the mercury ions[10] penetrate the
blood brain barrier and accumulate in the brain.[11] I believe this additional burden to my immune system was the
reason my health failed again, but on the other hand, I
could not have recovered without correcting my digestive
process.

(The Environmental Protection Agency has now made
paint manufacturers discontinue using mercury in their
latex products, but mercury-impregnated paint will still be
on the market for a while. To be safe, buy only latex paint
manufactured after January 1, 1991.)

My homeopathic physician was brilliant and obviously
saved my life, but mercury antidoted his remedy (prescription), and further improvement in me ceased.[12] Homeopathic physicians,[13] naturopathic doctors,[14] acu-
puncturists, and Chinese herbologists have a great deal
more to contribute to the healing process of chronic disease than the traditional medical community realizes.

Please keep in mind that each specialist tends to treat
symptoms from his own point of reference. They all frequently fail to recognize that it usually takes all three
specialists—a dental detoxicologist, an orthomolecular
psychiatrist or physician, and a clinical ecologist—to effec-
tively treat Alzheimer's disease or schizophrenia. You
would not expect to milk a cow while sitting on a one-
legged milking stool; you might wind up sitting in a cow-
pie. Similarly, it takes all three medical specialties—and a
lot of hard work on your part—to recover from Alzheimer's.

In the fifth edition of *Pharmacologic Principles of*

Medical Practice, authors John C. Krantz, Jr., and C. Jelleff Carr state:

> Chronic mercury poisoning may occur in individuals exposed to mercury compounds in industry. Absorption symptoms in the individual may present a misleading clinical picture. Mental and central nervous symptoms may be encountered in persons exposed to daily inhalation of mercury vapor.

I suspect the body might shut off stomach acid to prevent the absorption of deadly methyl mercury from silver fillings. Whatever the cause, a deficiency in stomach acid has been associated with anemia and allergies. According to *Remington's Pharmaceutical Sciences:*

> Glutamic Acid Hydrochloric is administered orally to counterbalance a deficiency of hydrochloric acid in the gastric juices, and to inhibit the growth of putrefactive microorganisms in ingested food. A deficiency of HCl [hydrochloric acid] is often associated with pernicious anemia, gastric carcinoma, congenital achlorhydria, and allergy.

Many other metals regularly used in dentistry, particularly nickel, may also cause autoimmune diseases such as arthritis, amyotrophic lateral sclerosis (Lou Gehrig's disease), lupus erythematosus, multiple sclerosis, Parkinson's disease, and some forms of cancer, according to *Candida, Silver (Mercury) Fillings and the Immune System,* by Betsy Russell Manning. A gentleman on his death bed kindly edited this manuscript in an early stage. He told me he did not believe that amalgam fillings could be the cause of the cancer he was expecting to die from shortly.

His gums, however, became so diseased that most of his teeth fell out, and thankfully, he recovered from his cancer.

I wish the clinical-ecology provocative-appraisal technique would be required as part of the test protocol for any new dental material before approval for distribution to the public. Also, I wish skeptical ADA-executive-board members, dental-school deans, and amalgam manufacturers wishing to prove the safety and efficacy of amalgam-filling materials would participate in provocative amalgam restoration tests—on themselves—within a hospital clinical ecology unit, controlled entirely by clinical ecologists. It would probably take less than three weeks out of their lives, and the results would end all speculation forever.

As you can see, the symptoms of mercury toxicity are many and varied. No one has all the symptoms, and no two people have the same set of symptoms. In addition, many symptoms may signal problems other than mercury toxicity. Do **not** diagnose yourself. If you suspect mercury toxicity, see your preferred health-care practitioner. Discuss with him (or her) all your suspicions and options.

In the rest of this chapter, I will discuss some of the options available, including the one that I chose.

GETTING RID OF THE CULPRITS

It took eleven years from the time my thinking process started deteriorating for me to find Dr. Huggins' book *It's All in Your Head*. This was the piece of the Alzheimer's puzzle that had been missing for so many wasted years.

An important word of caution: Do not attempt to have your amalgam fillings removed before carefully reading *It's All in Your Head*. If you are ill enough to need this book, then your amalgam fillings *must* be removed in a specific sequential order. (For a further discussion of the importance of proper amalgam removal and replacement, see Chapter Six of this book.) If there is ever a time for you to be in charge of your treatment procedures, it is now. If your dentist refuses to follow these *exact* procedures, *get up from his chair and walk out.* Telephone Dr. Huggins (see Appendix C) and find a dentist in your area who will comply with the procedures. Otherwise, you may be permanently injured.

Remember that you, not your dentist, are ultimately in charge of your health (and pocketbook). Be sure to use the proper replacement or removal sequence and vitamin therapy, and check for biocompatibility of the new filling materials by either working through Dr. Huggins, who does blood tests, or through a physician who is familiar with the Voll Electro-acupuncture Machine.

I decided to have all my teeth removed and to have this done by an oral surgeon. Fortunately, the surgeon used panorex (dental x-ray) equipment[15] that revealed six amalgam fragments: four small pieces within my gum tissue and two larger pieces approximately a half-inch down in my jawbone. (See Figure 2.1, on page 42.) Fragments are pieces of amalgam that were not cleaned up during dental treatment and worked their way into the oral cavity. They can lodge anywhere. Make sure additional panorex are taken after all your fillings or teeth are removed. Half of my amalgam fragments were found during this stage. Two additional minuscule fragments were found a year later.

I had realized all of the amalgam in my jaw was not completely cleaned up because a patch of skin high on my arm remained slightly blotchy and scabby. My oral surgeon increased the intensity of the x-ray machine slightly and found the two additional fragments. What surprised everyone was that one of the fragments, the deepest of all within my jawbone, was no larger than the point of a pin.

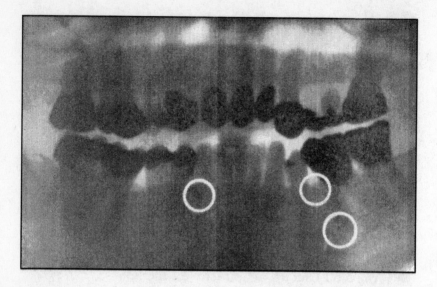

Figure 2.1.   The panorex (dental x-ray) that revealed the six
amalgam fragments lodged in my gums and jaw-
bone. Three of the pieces (circled) can be clearly
identified.

The oral surgeon, his assistant, and I could all barely see
it.

One reason some people do not recover after amalgam
replacement is that some amalgam fragments might be
remaining within their oral cavity. It is up to the dental
patient to check his x-rays until he is completely satisfied
that every single piece of fragment has been removed.
Another reason people do not recover completely is that
they forget the "other two legs of the milking stool." We
will discuss the other two medical specialties in Chapters 3
and 4.

A dental laboratory advised me to require that my new
false teeth be slowly dried at a low temperature over a
period of at least eleven hours to allow the monomers and
polymers to be released from the plates. Dental lab tech-

nicians like to cut the drying time, which may cause your mouth to blister or bum due to an allergic reaction to the monomers and polymers. Polymers and monomers are also released if dental plates are dried in a vacuum.

In addition to monomers and polymers in dental plates in general, mercury is also sometimes found in dental plates that are colored pink. It is in the pink dye. According to Dr. Huggins, it is always a good idea to have your plates made from a clear plastic material.[16]

The new composite filling materials that I tried before undergoing biocompatibility testing caused me to have severe swelling reactions for about six weeks. Voll Electroacupuncture Machine testing indicated there were not enough biocompatible dental filling materials available to warrant the replacement of my existing fillings. At the time I had my dental work completed, serum biocompatibility procedures were just in the process of being developed.

Dr. Huggins insists that everyone should undergo serum biocompatibility testing to determine their subsequent material selection. Other testing procedures do not allow the actual immuno observation of corrosives in relation to substitute filling materials.

Two dentists I visited refused to remove my teeth—that is, until I accidentally broke a very old bridge. As the dentist removed a large amount of silver amalgam from beneath the gold crown supporting one side of the bridge, something—I don't know words to adequately describe the sensation, although Dr. Huggins says "it was electricity"—instantly relaxed within my brain directly above the bridge. The same sensation was repeated several weeks later on the opposite side of my brain when the largest piece of amalgam fragment was surgically removed from my jawbone.

When the oral surgeon returned my gold-filled teeth

for my disposition, I broke the filling material loose. Amalgam and copper traces were found under most of the gold
crowns.

The brain allergies that nearly killed me are now just a
minor nuisance. Scabs and sores on my arms, which Dr.
Huggins says were caused by mercury and copper leaching from my silver fillings, quickly disappeared after
being a problem for almost fifty years. Homeopathic physicians have told me that the body sends disease and
pollution as far away from the major organs as possible—
to the skin. I believe them.

WILMA'S STORY

Wilma is a family friend who is a psychiatric nurse. After
reviewing this book, she told me that her mother, who had
been a schoolteacher, had cautioned her never to have a
bridge placed in her mouth. Her mother had told her that
after she had had a bridge installed, she became agitated,
cranky, and nervous, and could not sleep well at night.

Later, Wilma's mother had had her teeth removed, and
her symptoms vanished. She would point out people in
church who had recently had their teeth pulled and say,
"Now, you watch." Sure enough, within six months, they,
too, got rosy cheeks and felt better. Her mother used to
ask people who were having emotional problems, "How's
your teeth?"

At that time, it was known that dental cavities poisoned
the system, but the cavities themselves—not the silver
fillings—were suspected of being the cause of illness. Iron-
ically, research literature indicates that for more than 160
years, many dentists believed amalgam was bioincompatible. However, dentists concerned about the toxicity of
mercury within silver fillings were literally outlawed by
the American Dental Association.

In 1980, my dentist told me that less than 5 percent of the population has problems with mercury. And as the toxicity of silver-amalgam fillings began to be publicized, he lowered the figure to only one percent. That conservative estimate, however, still comes to more than 2.6 million people in the United States. Since then, I have been told, in private, by dentists, microbiologists, and immunologists who do blood serum tests that the one-percent figure is preposterous. Some dental toxicologists have found up to 68 percent of their patients sensitive to mercury, which suggests that the actual figure in the United States might be closer to 80–100 million people. A dentist once telephoned me from across the United States to tell me that he cried like a baby when he realized what he had done to his patients.

Amalgam fillings should be called by the name of the largest amount of metal within them: silver fillings should be called "mercury fillings." The misnomer is a deliberate deception to keep the public unaware that the dental profession has been placing a deadly poison directly into our bodies.

If you have a chronic disease and your dentist insists on using silver-amalgam filling material, find another dentist familiar with Dr. Huggins' procedures. Your chronic disease may not need to be chronic.

OTHER FILLING MATERIALS

Mercury is not the only dental filling material that is controversial. Two others are copper and aluminum.

Copper

In the northwest, where I live, there has been so much controversy in the local newspapers recently over amalgam fillings that area dentists are beginning to use what they call "high-copper fillings." High-copper fillings are supposed to contain less mercury. However, copper itself is a problem because it enhances galvanic action in the oral cavity.

In 1972, the National Institute for Occupational Safety and Health (NIOSH) set the maximum copper level allowed in silver fillings at 6 percent. And yet, the new high-copper fillings contain as much as 30 percent. In addition, high-copper fillings are so much more reactive galvanically that they emit methyl mercury at a rate fifty times faster than conventional amalgams.

Aluminum

Six years ago, a microbiology professor told my son that although microbiologists couldn't prove it (at the time), they believed beer and cola drinks leach aluminum ions off aluminum beverage containers. These ions, they believed, are then absorbed into the brains of some Alzheimer's patients.

Recently, Dr. Huggins had a patient who exhibited very high levels of aluminum toxicity. He found that the patient drank six cans of beer every night. Dr. Huggins told the man to drink bottled beer. Within a short time, the man's aluminum levels returned to normal.

Several of my mother's old aluminum cooking pots were deeply pitted. The acid in a stewing tomato will clean an aluminum pot, but the tomato itself will stew your brain with the aluminum. Do not use aluminum cooking utensils, baking-powder biscuits, underarm deodorants, antacid pills containing aluminum, or aluminum oxygen canisters. Check all labels!

Some of the new resin dental fillings are a composite of more than twenty different materials, including aluminum. The base of some porcelain crowns is aluminum. If you do not know all the elements within a proposed dental composite, use the Voll system or blood tests to determine biocompatibility. Your mouth is an acid environment, and according to Dr. Jeffrey Bland, author of *Your Health Under Siege,* aluminum is readily absorbed into the brain if you have any degree of calcium deficiency.

REMOVING METALS FROM THE REST OF THE BODY

After you have removed the metal from your mouth, you will also need to remove the metals from the rest of your body. Combinations of amino acids and minerals are available at health-food stores and from Dr. Huggins' office to accomplish this. First, have your hair, blood, and urine tested to determine your specific toxicities.

Homeopathic remedies to remove mercury and lead seemed to work very well for me. They drove the metal that had accumulated within my body directly to my skin. Small black particles appeared on my skin under my heart in a shot-gun pattern with a circumference about the size of a coffee-can lid. But remember: this procedure will not work if any silver fillings or fragments are still in your mouth. The mercury in your blood will return to its former level.

While taking your homeopathic remedy, do not forget to take vitamin and mineral supplements to replenish the necessary elements.

After you have replaced all your bioincompatible fillings, allow your body nine or ten months to rid itself of mercury. If your body does not respond satisfactorily— and you have diligently followed Dr. Huggins' directions, plus rechecked for amalgam fragments—consider ethylene diamine tetraacetic acid (EDTA) chelation therapy, which will complete the withdrawal of heavy metals from your body.[17]

Autopsies have revealed excess mercury, aluminum, copper, and lead in the brain of Alzheimer's and schizophrenia patients, so I had extensive EDTA treatment five years ago. It was not effective, however, because unknown to both my physician and me, mercury was continually leaching from my amalgam fillings.

A MIXTURE OF METALS ACTING TOGETHER

Although we never think of it as such, vitality—that wonderful abundance of energy, the sparkle in the eyes, the bounce in the step, and the smile on the face—is actually caused by electricity. If you don't believe this, try living without it. If the electricity stops in your body, you're dead.

Homeopathic physicians and many dentists know that the electricity generated by galvanic reactions to amalgam fillings can pass from one side of a dental bridge, up into the brain, and then down again through the opposite bridge abutment to complete an unending circle of electrical interruption of the vitality. Homeopathic physicians say that disease can only manifest itself when the body's electromagnetic field, which flows throughout the entire body along definite pathways, is disturbed. Furthermore, the higher the electrical current is that is generated by the dissimilar metals within the oral cavity, the faster methyl mercury is released and absorbed into the body. And on top of everything else, mercury destroys DNA within the cells.

A story in the December 1990 issue of *Health Consciousness* magazine entitled "Gaston Naessens: Discoverer of the Somatid," by Christopher Bird, suggests that certain minuscule life forms are imperishable. "At the death of their hosts," Bird says, "they return to the earth—where they live on for thousands, or millions, perhaps billions of years . . . the cycle we've discovered adds up to no less than a brand new understanding for the very basis of life." In 1944, R. E. Seidel, a homeopathic physician, was convinced from his studies that "germs could not be the cause, but are the result of disease . . . that cells, regarded as the irreducible building blocks of living matter, are actually composed of smaller cells, themselves made up of even smaller cells, etc." I believe that the end stage of what these scientists have discovered will turn out to be electricity.

Sometimes the galvanic reaction between my gold crowns and silver fillings was so strong that I thought it could illuminate a flashlight! A galvanic reaction can produce up to one thousand times more electricity than the brain is capable of handling. Dr. Huggins believes that the brain short-circuiting has probably caused over 50 percent of the neurological diseases in the patients he has been seeing. He reports that more than 90 percent of his patients with epilepsy show improvement following the removal of their fillings. Galvanic current was also the source of my heart irregularities, which vanished after I had all the metal removed from my mouth.

As you can see, metal—especially mercury—toxicity can very well be a major factor in many illnesses, especially Alzheimer's disease, schizophrenia, and neurological diseases such as multiple sclerosis. Having all your teeth pulled may be a drastic remedy, but having all your fillings changed is not, especially since fillings only have a limited lifespan and most people need them replaced periodically anyway.

In Chapter 3, we will look at the second leg of the milking stool: allergies.

3.

Allergies, Allergies Everywhere

The science of one generation is usually the fallacy of the next.

—Sir Arthur Conan Doyle
English author

Allergies have been called the "twentieth-century illness." They are a reaction to a myriad of substances: chemical sprays, hydrocarbons, environmental pollutants, foreign substances in water, pollens, and foods, to name a few. And the pollutants, as well as the allergies, are becoming more and more prevalent. My physicians have told me, for instance, that I am what the whole population three generations away will be like if we refuse to clean up the environment.

So, the second book on our must-read list is *An Alternative Approach to Allergies*, by Dr. Theron Randolph. Read about chemical susceptibilities and the pollution all around us, then begin avoiding synthesized chemicals in all forms as much as possible. Next, list your ten favorite foods—the foods you cannot do without. *Do without them,* in all forms, for at least ten days. Check all food labels. If you start feeling really lousy during this ten-day period, you may have food, chemical, or pollen allergies. Read and study all the allergy books on the must-read list.

In the meantime, however, read this chapter. In it, I will give you a brief run-down of the major allergens, including environmental pollutants, hydrocarbons, pollens, and Candida. Then I will discuss the major ways to combat them.

THE VARIOUS CAUSES OF ALLERGIES

There are many causes of allergies today. Almost everything in the world is an allergen to someone. Some allergens are more common than others, however. The following are the most common for Alzheimer's victims.

Environmental Pollutants

The chemical-contamination cycle is seen most clearly in nature. The waters of Puget Sound next to Washington State's major cities are cesspools. A cannery in Anacortes, Washington, refused to process salmon caught near Seattle because the fish were soft and unappetizing. A woman discovered a young cougar dead near a stream deep within a forest. In trying to find the cause of the animal's death, she discovered that its liver was as hard as a rock. She found dead trout, like those the cougar had been eating, floating in the stream, and upon examination, found that many had tumors. She attributed the diseases in both the fish and cougar to the chemicals used by the local timber companies. Do not assume that wild meat is uncontaminated.

My family and I used to see dear friends in Ashford, Washington, outside the southwestern entrance to Mount

Rainier. We loved to visit the area and always entered the park through Ashford. Then we read that seven expectant mothers had miscarriages after the timber companies applied chemicals to their company-owned forest lands outside the park. We decided to stay away for a while.

Three years later, we visited Ashford again. Several restaurants there offer delicious wild-blackberry pie, which we had been looking forward to. We stopped at a restaurant, and I asked the waitress where all the deer and bears had gone. We used to see them near the park entrance. The waitress looked puzzled. "You know, I haven't seen them for about three years now," she said. "What will you have?" We ordered tomato juice and left.

Whenever chemicals are sprayed around your living area, you should take the following precautions:

- Wash off your boots and walkway so you don't track the chemicals into your house and onto your carpet.
- If pregnant, do not mow the lawn. In fact, to be safe, stay off the grass completely for a while.
- Keep pets indoors. If you need to put them outdoors, leave them out for at least a few days before bringing them back in. Then check their skin for rashes, which may indicate toxic chemical exposure, and give them a hose-down and lukewarm bath.

Allergy patients (universal reactors) are always looking for an uncontaminated area in which to live. I am no exception. I once drove to Mount Baker, in northwestern Washington, through a town named Bellingham. I had been wondering if the area northeast of Bellingham and up to the Canadian border might be remote enough to be an environmental oasis. It turned out to be beautiful dairy-farm country, but the chemical manufacturers are ubiquitous: so many farmers were spraying their fields, I developed burning brain sensations that I had not had in three years.

A helicopter-pilot friend of mine quit a high-paying job spraying wheat fields in eastern Washington because the insecticide he used was so potent that contact with a cut, such as one that he would get in a crash, could mean death in fourteen to sixteen hours. No one on Earth would be able to save him, he said.

The Northwest Healing Arts Center, of Bellevue, Washington, says there are over 70,000 chemical combinations that have been produced and used in the United States, including 7,000 toxic chemicals still in daily use. Senator Patrick Leahy, of Vermont, chairman of the Senate Agriculture Committee, has indicated that he intends to investigate the potential dangers from chemicalized food. He believes the scales have been tipped in favor of agricultural chemicals, making them a liability to our health and environment. Toxins in the food chain appear to be more harmful than the general population knows. Clinical ecologists have been trying to warn us for many years about the dangerous chemical toxins in the food chain that cause chronic illness.

I once met a hospitalized Mexican farm laborer who stuffed cotton in his ears and nose, and wore goggles and a bandanna over his mouth. No one suspected that agricultural chemicals were the source of his psychotic behavior. Sometimes the schizophrenic behavior itself provides clues to the root cause of the psychosis, as well as to the most beneficial treatment process, which in this particular case should have been chemical detoxification and vitamin therapy instead of psychoanalysis.

The United Farm Workers of America (UFWA) claims that hundreds of thousands of farm workers and their children are poisoned by toxic pesticides every year. It says that one-third of all pesticides cause cancer and that some of these pesticides will not wash off under the kitchen tap. The organization is currently endeavoring to have what it considers the five most dangerous—captan, parathion, phosdrin, dinoseb, and methyl bromide—withdrawn from use in fields. (See Appendix C on how to order a videotape describing the group's effort.)

The Foundation for Advancement in Science and Education (FASE) says that the problem is not confined to the United States. According to an article in its Winter/Spring 1991 publication:

> The World Health Organization (WHO) estimated approximately 3 million cases of pesticide poisoning were occurring annually, with approximately 220,000 deaths. This year WHO estimated that as many as 25 million agricultural workers in the developing world suffer an episode of pesticide poisoning each year.

The FASE article continues with a claim that should make Americans in particular take notice:

> Literally billions of pounds of pesticides which have been determined to be unsafe in this country are being shipped to foreign ports. More than 6,075 tons of pesticides classified as extremely toxic, including cancelled compounds such as mirex, heptachlor and chlordane, were shipped to such countries as Guatemala, Brazil, Sri Lanka and scores of other foreign ports. An additional 2,750 tons known or suspected to be mutagens or carcinogens or that could cause reproductive or prenatal effects were shipped.

What is not recognized by Americans is that these pesticides come back to us in the products we purchase from those countries. As an example, the Environmental Protection Agency (EPA) banned a certain chemical manufactured in California from all use in this country. The Agency for International Development then stepped in and bought the entire batch, shipping it to Brazil. The company had so much success with the chemical that it eventually built a plant of its own in a third-world country to manufacture the pesticide and ship it out to other third-world countries. The chemical then came back to the United States from Brazil on the coffee imported from Brazil.

Hydrocarbons

Many allergies are related to petroleum products. During an accidental exposure to auto exhaust fumes in a clinical ecology hospital unit, I "saw" my fingers separate from my hand and move slightly sideways. I also seemed to be able to see the floor through the separations.

Petroleum fumes are quickly disabling to a potential Alzheimer's victim. If you must drive, use an automobile air cleaner, such as Foust 160-A. Otherwise, you may run into severe problems before your vitamin-and-mineral therapy has a chance to reverse the disease process. It took me approximately four months of taking vitamins and, in particular, trace minerals before I noticed any improvement in my ability to tolerate petroleum fumes on the freeway, along with a few other chemical odors elsewhere.

I remember a hospitalized mental patient who was sent home twenty-three times. He showed no indication of mental distress while in the hospital, but he always became schizophrenic and had to be returned to the hospital within five days. That was many years ago and the patient is most likely deceased by now, but I would give ten-to-one odds that his home-heating system used petroleum products.

I am also reminded of a nun who had all kinds of medical problems. Finally, she mentioned to her family physician that she lit a candle in her room every evening and prayed for her health to improve.

A woman who did all her cooking and heating with an old-fashioned wood-and-coal stove that smoked had schizophrenia for forty years. Her schizophrenia went into remission after she moved into an apartment that had electric baseboard heating.

I could go on.

Wood stoves, fireplaces, oil, gas, diesel, propane, candles, ink in newspapers and books, floor wax, and furniture polish all "out-gas" hydrocarbon fumes. Hydrocarbon fumes cause severe brain-fog reactions in the majority of people who notice cerebral allergic reactions to other substances.

Books can present a particularly annoying problem, especially when you're trying to learn what you can do to combat your Alzheimer's or other problems. One solution I have found involves baking soda. Sprinkle baking soda (using a large salt shaker to make it easy) onto the pages of a new book to get rid of the hydrocarbon smell, then set the book aside for a few days. Add more baking soda, if necessary. When the hydrocarbon smell is neutralized, blow away the soda from the book with a vacuum cleaner set in reverse. In the summer, open all new books wide and place them in a protected area outside to air out for several days.

If your furnace or garage are *under* your house, change your heating system to electricity and do not park your car in the garage. Gas fumes rise. They'll rise into your house. The only way you can use a gas heating system is to put the furnace apart and downwind from the house. Place the vent on the roof of the building housing the furnace and face the fresh-air intake into the wind, on the opposite side from the exhaust vent, about four feet off the ground. Place a filter over the fresh-air intake to remove gas, chemicals, and pollens. Then transfer the heat into your house by means of a heat exchanger. The inside air will be exchanged every hour. The system works very well, but you must still do all your cooking on an *electric* stove.

Electromagnetic Fields

Dr. Leonard Sagan, a physician working with the utility-sponsored Electric Power Research Institute, of Palo Alto, California, says there is growing evidence that ordinary electricity may be a health hazard. This, naturally, is an increasing worry for power-industry executives,[1] which prompted the electric industry to provide $2.5 million for low-level electromagnetic-radiation (EMR) research in 1987.

Computer monitors have been called the "asbestos of the nineties." I developed depression and short-term memory loss every time I turned on my computer and had to delay working on this book for many months before IBM scientists finally acknowledged there might be a problem. American monitors release substantially higher amounts of low-level radiation than is permitted in Europe. IBM consultants eventually advised me to purchase a Sun-Flex mesh radiation cover (see Appendix D), which reduces approximately 95 percent of the radiation emitted from a screen and, happily, also reduces the glare. The Washington State Patrol has also placed radiation screens on all of its computer monitors. Findings show that a secretary who uses a monitor cover is less tired, more accurate, and more productive.

IBM has now lowered the radiation level on its new Model 8515 computer monitor to meet Swedish standards. The monitor is a pleasure to use, but after checking, I decided to get another Sun-Flex screen anyway. My desk is too small to move the monitor as far away from me as I would like.

To determine how close you can safely sit to a particular monitor, cover a portable radio with aluminum foil, leaving only the receiver free. Punch a tiny hole in the foil at the speaker. Find a point between stations, turn the volume up as high as it will go, and place the radio close to the monitor. Then slowly withdraw the radio from the monitor until the static disappears. The point where the static disappears is the closest you should sit to the monitor. With most monitors, this is approximately thirty-six inches. (While we're on the subject, keep the kids—and yourself—at least six feet back from a nineteen-inch television screen.)

There is evidence that the electromagnetic radiation from household appliances may be the newest threat to the body's ability to fight disease and regulate its immune system. My homeopathic physician, Dr. Dean Crothers, told me several years ago not to use electric blankets because they zap your strength. Clinical ecologists have told me not to use electric blankets because the heat from the electric wire causes the plastic covering on the wire to emit plastic fumes, which cause brain-fog reactions.

Water

The EPA has identified 900 inert ingredients in pesticides that it has no information on. In California, 57 pesticides have contaminated more than 2,500 wells, according to research reported to the California Legislative Assembly. An additional 1,400 wells were found unfit for any use.

Iowa researchers discovered more than 400 public water systems to have pesticide contamination in the drinking water.

The *San Francisco Examiner* reports that there is so much chlorine in water, some sensitive individuals cannot take showers without suffering skin rashes, stuffiness, and headaches. Until I purchased a Cuno AP-600 filter with a 617 chlorine cartridge, I could not even walk into the bathroom or laundry room, or run the kitchen tap. Severe brain-fog reactions caused my personality to change drastically within just five minutes. I have been pleased with my Cuno filtering system. It's a good product for removing chlorine from the whole house. However, all cartridge-type filters back up enough toxins to eventually leach the chemicals back into the drinking water. Change the filter often.

The Rain Crystal Pyrex glass distiller for the secondary treatment of drinking water at the point of use is recommended by Jim Nigra, who is the most knowledgeable and helpful environmental purification expert I have found anywhere. The Skagit County Public Utility District had placed a full-page ad in Washington State newspapers (see Figure 3.1) during the summer of 1988 indicating that lead was leaching from water pipes, so I ordered the distiller for my home. Keep in mind, however, that you will need to take mineral supplements and eat lots of salads if you use a distiller because it also distills good minerals. You will know you need mineral supplementation if your hair becomes like wire and you develop ridges running lengthwise on your fingernails.

Pollens

During spring allergy season, pollens can cause symptoms ranging from a vague, unpleasant feeling that something is

WHAT THE EPA SAYS ABOUT LEAD IN YOUR DRINKING WATER

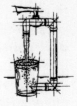

The United States Environmental Protection Agency (EPA) sets drinking water standards and has determined that lead is a health concern at certain levels of exposure There is currently a standard of 50 parts per billion (ppb) Based on new health information, EPA is likely to lower this standard significantly. ("Fifty parts per billion" is like one drop in 180 gallons)

Part of the purpose of this notice is to inform you of the potential adverse health effects of lead This is being done even though your water may not be in violation of the current standard

EPA and others are concerned about lead in drinking water Too much lead in the human body can cause serious damage to the brain, kidneys, nervous system, and red blood cells The greatest risk, even with short term exposure, is to young children and pregnant women

WHAT IS LEAD?

Lead is a heavy, soft gray metal which is harmful to human health if inhaled or swallowed Lead from automobile exhaust and from industry are the major sources of lead contamination

HOW DOES LEAD GET INTO YOUR BODY?

Lead enters the body through food, air and water. For most people, the major source of lead is from food. Drinking water contributes about 10 to 20 percent of the average person's lead intake. Other ways lead many enter the body include:

* Dust, soil, or food grown near busy roadways
* Certain soldered food cans, especially sour foods such as fruit or saurkraut
* Imported pottery, antique cookware and pottery
* Surface preparation before painting
* Lead paint chips
* Colored newsprint
* Various hobbies or jobs which use lead solder, weights, or ammunition
* Folk remedies such as <u>Azarcon</u> or <u>greta</u> contain up to 90 percent lead

Information on how to measure lead content in a sample of paint, dust or ceramic dishware can be obtained through the PUD Your physician can measure levels of lead in blood.

<u>Lead is of special concern for infants, toddlers, and young children because of their immature nervous systems.</u> An amount of lead that would have little effect on an adult can have a big effect on a small body Youngsters are also at risk because they put things in their mouth which may contain lead <u>Pregnant women are of particular concern</u> because too much lead could injure their unborn babies.

COULD LEAD BE IN YOUR DRINKING WATER?

In Washington State, lead does not appear to be a problem at the source where the water originates However, it can be a concern at the faucet because <u>water can pick up lead from the household plumbing system.</u> Not all homeowners need to be concerned about lead in their drinking water Lead levels in your home drinking water are likely to be highest:

* If your home or water system has lead pipes, or
* If your home has copper pipes with lead solder, and
  - If the home is less than five years old, or
  - If you have soft or acidic water, or
  - If water sits in the pipes for several hours

The only way to know for sure if lead is present in household water is to have it tested by a laboratory approved by the Department of Social and Health Services (DSHS). This should involve two tests: a "first draw" sample and a fully flushed sample They cost between $11 and $20 per test Even if you use a home filtering device, you should still be concerned about lead in your drinking water The PUD has a list of approved laboratories within Northwest Washington for you.

HOW TO REDUCE LEAD IN YOUR DRINKING WATER

Lead levels in air and food have been significantly lowered since 1977 thanks to concerned health officials and EPA regulations If your plumbing contains lead, or if your drinking water is found to contain high levels of lead, here are some simple actions which can reduce the lead:

* Use water from the cold water tap for drinking, cooking and making baby formula Hot tap water may contain higher levels of lead than cold tap water
* If building or remodeling, use plastic pipes or copper pipes joined with lead-free solder Lead-free solder is now required by law
* Support building officials in their effort to eliminate lead solder in new plumbing.
* If your water has not been used for several hours, "flush your faucet" for about two or three minutes You may choose to save this water for future use such as watering your plants
* One you have "flushed your faucet", fill a clean pitcher and keep it in the refrigerator for later use

WHAT THE PUBLIC UTILITY DISTRICT IS DOING TO HELP

The District has begun construction of a new water treatment plant which will not only filter water but make it less likely to pick up lead from your plumbing system. Every effort will be taken to complete the project by fall of 1989. Meanwhile, ways to make the District's water even less corrosive will continue to be evaluated.

IF YOU REQUIRE FURTHER INFORMATION

If you have questions about lead in your drinking water, or if you wish a list of laboratories that will test for lead, call Public Utility District No 1 of Skagit County, 424-7104. Specific questions can be directed to Greg Peterka.

EPA has provided the public with a toll free number for more information on lead Their number is 1-800-426-4791 The State Health Department (DSHS) will also have a toll free number 1-800-521-0323 after mid-June The Skagit County Health Department is available to answer questions on lead Their number is 336-9380 If you have questions about your health and lead, talk to your physician

This information has been provided to you as a public service by Skagit PUD

Figure 3.1.   The newspaper advertisement placed by the Skagit County Public Utility District.

not quite right to acute brain-fog reactions. They caused many unpleasant cerebral reactions in me, including severe depression, acute brain fog, and burning brain sensations.

If you have burning sensations in your brain and suspect pollens are the cause, you need a Dustfoe 66 or 77 mask with filters, available from Mine Safety Appliances (see Appendix D). The masks are really designed for dust, but allergy patients find that they work better than any mask designed for pollens. These masks, however, are not designed for chemicals.

In addition to a mask, get a stainless steel room air filter and find a clinical ecologist. The sooner you do these things, the better your chances are of avoiding the final stages of irreversible brain damage.

Candida Albicans

The third book on the must-read list is *The Yeast Connection: A Medical Breakthrough*, by William G. Crook, M.D. Candida overgrowth is a yeast infection that indicates the immune system is exhausted. Notice that in nature, mold does not grow on young, healthy forest trees. Fresh vegetables and fruits never have mold. The Candida-overgrowth–mental-health connection is not generally known to the psychiatric and medical communities. The first book on the subject—*The Missing Diagnosis*, by C. Orian Truss, M.D.—was not published until 1983.

The signs of Candida overgrowth include an aversion to odors, premenstrual syndrome (PMS), depression, a nasty disposition, brain fog, and exhaustion after a full night's sleep. A disinterest in sex is also often noticed but quickly responds to a low-carbohydrate (60 grams) diet. (*Caution:* If porphyria psychosis has been diagnosed in any member of your family, even a distant relative, do not go on a high-protein–low-carbohydrate diet. Psychiatric symptoms may appear, according to Dr. Chris Reading, author of *Your Family Tree Connection*.

Every PMS victim should be tested for Candida overgrowth by her gynecologist. To do this, take a little Nystatin powder, an antifungal medication, on a toothpick in a glass of water. If you do not have a reaction within a half-hour, try a quarter teaspoon of Nystatin. If your symptoms do increase, you have a Candida overgrowth infection. You also, very likely, have a vitamin and mineral deficiency—and, possibly, a silver-filling problem—but you do *not* have a psychiatric problem. Candida overgrowth causes mental symptoms, as well as a host of other medical complaints. If you're sick and tired of being sick and tired, *The Yeast Connection* is an important book to read.

Candida can be a very difficult infection to get rid of. When attacked, it encapsulates within a protein shell and remains there until the immune system runs down again. It then continues on as before. Caprystatin and Capricin, two other antifungal medications, contain fatty acids that break down the protein shell and kill the Candida. However, I would prefer to start with Nizoral for ten days, then switch to Capricin, combined with one-eighth of a teaspoon of Nystatin, every four hours around the clock for approximately three months. Several members of my allergy groups have indicated that Nystatin powder alone is also effective in killing Candida in the alimentary tract, at a dose of one-eighth teaspoon six times a day.

Some physicians like to keep their patients on Nystatin for two or three years, but Nystatin is expensive. In addition, I was unable to control my Candida overgrowth until I began supplementing my Nystatin with hydrochloric acid and digestive enzymes according to my Heidelberg test results. Your physician should be able to advise you about this. If he is not familiar with Candida overgrowth infections, show him this section, or check with an allergy group in your area to find a physician who does understand the Candida treatment process. If your physician is interested in learning about Candida and its treatment, Dr. Crook will send him a free copy of *The Yeast Connection* (see Appendix C for the address of the International Health Foundation).

There are many causes of Candida overgrowth. The major culprit seems to be the indiscriminate use of antibiotics.[2] Some of the others are oral sex, sugar, junk food diets, steroids, stress, and birth control pills.

Odors

An acute aversion to odors indicates Candida overgrowth, according to *The Yeast Connection*. According to *Orthomolecular Medicine for Physicians*, by Dr. Abram Hoffer and Dr. Morton Walker, an acute aversion to odors also indicates low trace-mineral levels. If something smells unpleasant to you, move away from it, or move it away from you. Smells are a sign that something is out-gassing.

Many afflicted people do not notice the odors around them because their environment is so contaminated that they can't distinguish all the individual smells. We usually lose our sensitivity to an odor within twenty-four hours, even though it may continue to cause an adverse cerebral or physical reaction. For example, while men with Candida overgrowth cannot tolerate the smell of perfume, afflicted women who apply it liberally may not notice it at all. Many afflicted people who smoke heavily do not notice how much tobacco smoke stinks. Other odorous items in the environment that we may become used to are computers, printers, copy machines, toilets, shower and drinking water, soaps, and dust, to name just a few.

Mineral deficiencies can also interfere with the ability to smell an odor. According to Dr. Sandra Denton, the foremost mercury-chelation-therapy expert in the United States,[3] the lack of zinc can cause problems. Quite a few of the cerebral-allergy patients in my hospital clinical ecology unit were unable to detect the odors causing their distress. Luckily for them, however, during this time, I was hypersensitive to smells. The patients, therefore, used me (like a bloodhound, I guess) to sniff out the offending substances, and I was usually correct.

Be aware that mercury is often used in the tanning of leather for upholstery. If you are shopping for leather furniture, pass it by if it smells bad. If it doesn't smell bad, sit on it for a while to see if you react to it anyway. The symptoms often include itchy eyes and breathing problems. Dr. Randolph recommends that allergy sufferers buy cars that are at least two years old to allow time for all the chemical odors to evaporate. I, however, did not particularly notice a problem with my car, which has leather seats, when it was new.

I have been taking trace-mineral supplements for several years now, as suggested in *Orthomolecular Medicine for Physicians,* and many smells that formerly caused me to suffer severe brain-fog reactions—particularly petroleum fumes—have ceased being a problem. Other chemical fumes still cause mild brain fog, but I rarely think about petroleum fumes, dust, and pollens anymore.

Campylobacter Pyloritis

We have billions of friendly bacteria in our digestive system. *Campylobacter pyloritis* (CP) is not one of them. Both Candida and CP are signs of what is called the "leaky gut syndrome." The leaky gut syndrome is the suspected cause of many diseases.

Campylobacter pyloritis is considered to be the most important etiological factor in duodenal and peptic ulcers. It also often causes chronic nonspecific gastritis. Dr. Martin Lee, director of the Great Smokies Medical Laboratory, in Asheville, North Carolina, reports that healing has occurred in over 90 percent of his CP-infected ulcer patients when he treats them with bismuth preparations.

CP is additionally involved in food allergies, arthritis, Candida, and low stomach acid. Stomach acid will remain low until CP and Candida are eradicated. A bismuth citrate formula restored my stomach-acid production.

For more information on Campylobacter pyloritis and CP blood tests, contact the Great Smokies Medical Laboratory (see Appendix C).

Soap

Do **not** use perfumed or chlorinated laundry soap or scouring powder in any form! It will make you sick. I have found that Bon Ami is—by far—the best scouring powder available for allergic individuals. Palmolive makes an excellent unscented, hypoallergenic hand soap. Other hypoallergenic hand soaps and washing powders preferred by hypersensitive people are made by Lifetree and Ecover, and are sold in natural-food stores.

Until I had taken vitamins and minerals for approximately four months, the only soaps I was able to tolerate without a cerebral brain-fog reaction were Amway LOC in the shower and either Amway SA-8 or Arm and Hammer laundry powder for washing clothes. You might also find it necessary to rinse your laundry several times before drying it. For whitening, sodium hexametaphosphate substitutes very well for chlorine (see Appendix D for where to purchase).

Never store soaps, cleansers, chemicals, plastics, or

aluminum foil in your kitchen. Keep all scented and smelly items away from your living areas. I store my laundry soap in an outside storage shed. When I need some in the house, I fill a glass jar from the main container and keep it tightly sealed.

HOW TO COMBAT ALLERGIES

There is no one cure for Alzheimer's disease, schizophrenia, or most of the individual allergies discussed thus far in this chapter. There are, however, many little steps you can take to effect what might amount to a cure. We will discuss several of these steps in the rest of this chapter.

The Clean Room

Brain-fog, brain-fag, schizophrenia, and Alzheimer's sufferers must protect themselves from the environment long enough to recover sufficiently to allow the disease process to reverse itself. Every brain-fog victim requires what is called an "oasis"—an environmentally clean room, preferably a bedroom—in which to "crash" until his thinking clears. You will find it impossible to cooperate in your own treatment process, or to recover, without an oasis.

Keep your oasis aired out as much as possible. Strip it of everything—including the mattresses—and remove every item from the closet, especially wool clothes that have been dry-cleaned (hydrocarbons are used to dry-clean wool clothes). If you are not allergic to wool or cotton, you can leave blankets made of these materials. Challenge yourself by returning just one item to the room every night.

If a bathroom adjoins the room, keep the door closed. If the house in general is less than seven years old, or the carpet in your oasis is synthetic and less than five years old, formaldehyde may be a problem; testing kits are available by mail order (see Appendix D). Remove all synthetic, multicolored carpets that are less than ten years old; the more colors a synthetic carpet has, the more formaldehyde it has because every time a different color dye was added, the carpet was again dipped into that chemical. Natural-fiber carpets are fine—unless you're allergic to wool or cotton. Also remove all particle-board subflooring less than seven years old and all plasterboard finish, both of which have formaldehyde. If the heating system is a forced-air type, seal the bedroom air vents to keep out any air pollution from the other parts of the house. You will soon learn what else you should do.

Remove all books and newspapers from the house in general. Children are especially prone to allergies to ink. Store your books in sealed cardboard boxes on portable shelving positioned at least five inches from the wall to allow air circulation; leave a light on over the boxes in damp and cold weather to prevent mold. Bring only one book into the house at a time. Never place books on the table beside your bed.

If you live or work near a busy roadway, sell your house or change your job. Move at least three miles from a freeway. My family and I now live in a lovely small town by the sea where everyone from the city longs to vacation.

Detoxification

The organ that is primarily responsible for removing chemicals from the bloodstream is the liver. In turn, any toxins that the liver is unable to metabolize and dispose of quickly enough, it deposits as far away from the major organs as possible: in the fat tissues throughout the body, including the layer of fat beneath the skin. Many harmful metals, chemicals, and diseases are driven to, and removed from the body through, the skin. However, once

the liver and fat tissues are saturated, the toxins are released back into the bloodstream and reabsorbed by the
body.

Naturopathic physicians have told me that when the
blood is continually circulating chemicals—medical drugs,
street drugs, solvents, pesticides, herbicides—the body
cannot be healthy; the body is poisoned. They believe that
most cancers and autoimmune diseases, including rheumatoid arthritis and lupus, can be directly related to such
poisoning.

An allergic reaction to a minuscule amount of chemical
is a clear signal that the liver is overloaded from environmental contamination. The sufferer's system then experiences a reaction syndrome that physicians call a "chemical
sensitivity." Fortunately, an individual who is a "walking
toxic-waste dump" can remove most of the chemicals from
his body through a toxin-cleansing and tissue-restoration
program. One facility that offers such a program is the
Northwest Healing Arts Center, in Bellevue, Washington
(see Appendix C). A tissue-cleansing program was recommended to me by my clinical ecologist.

Plants

Dr. William Wolverton, of the National Space Tech-
nologies Laboratories, in Bay St. Louis, Mississippi, found
that a spider plant reduces the formaldehyde level in a
sealed chamber by 85 percent in twenty-four hours. Peace
lilies, Chinese evergreens, and golden pathos have the
same air-cleansing ability. They were also able to filter out
carbon monoxide and nitrogen dioxide. Dr. Wolverton
reports that three or four plants can continuously filter the
air in a twelve-by-fifteen-foot room.

Be very careful, however, not to overwater plants or
the soil may mold. In fact, if you suspect you have a
Candida-overgrowth infection, remove all plants from

your home until the Candida is killed, otherwise the mold will cause reactions.

There are excellent air cleaners available that remove formaldehyde, but plants can be an inexpensive solution.

Nutrition and Vitamin Therapy

My wife, who is a pharmacist, attended a seminar cosponsored by her company and a vitamin manufacturer. The speaker was the president of Health Media, publisher of *The Nutrition Report*. He reads over 800 articles on nutrition every month. Part of Louise's notes read:

Inadequate nutrition—subclinical symptoms

1. Impaired immune response
2. Adverse effects upon behavior
3. Reduced metabolism of drugs and environmental chemicals

Perhaps, in his book *Nutrition and Vitamin Therapy*, the fourth book on our must-read list, Dr. Michael Lesser expresses it best when he says, "Physicians need to recognize the sick patient is often a hungry and/or a chemically poisoned patient." He then gives scores of case histories to illustrate his point. Nothing I could write could teach you more about nutrition and vitamin therapy than Dr. Lesser's book. Another good teaching tool is *Pottenger's Cats*, by Dr. Francis F. Pottenger.

I find it interesting that my friend Bill Vaughn, from Spokane, Washington, recovered from Alzheimer's symptoms, crippling arthritis, and obesity by following a regimen of vitamins, minerals, and herbs. Bill then went to work for the company that makes the particular supplements he used. He is now helping other people with chronic and acute diseases who have made the traditional medical rounds without success.

In the fifth book on our must-read list, *Nutrients to Age Without Senility,* Dr. Abram Hoffer tells the story of some former Canadian prisoners-of-war who were starved during World War II and later developed schizophrenia. Doctors determined that their prolonged starvation depleted their vitamin and mineral reserves, which caused their mental distress. The former prisoners recovered and continued in excellent mental health *until they discontinued their vitamin therapy.* I have found this to be true for me, too.

Dr. Hoffer recommends niacin against Alzheimer's disease. I have found that time-release niacin works the best for me because I can tolerate the large dose of niacin without experiencing the strong flushing side effect of regular niacin. But no matter what form you take—nor what specific vitamins and minerals—if you have any sort of mental distress in your background, continue your vitamin therapy, particularly if it includes niacin and trace minerals, for the remainder of your life.

Niacin, as mentioned, is an important vitamin in the fight against Alzheimer's. It is also effective at lowering cholesterol and especially helpful in orthomolecular psychiatric treatment, but it often must be used in high doses to achieve results. Physicians caution their patients to be aware that high doses of niacin (vitamin B-3) can increase both blood sugar (a problem in diabetes) and uric acid (a problem with gout), and can activate peptic ulcers. Gout and peptic-ulcer reactions are noticed immediately, but blood-sugar reactions are not, so check your blood-sugar levels once in a while. Gout suggests the patient is not drinking enough water, so increase your intake of fluids. Gout and stomach pain additionally both indicate the need to immediately contact your physician, hopefully an orthomolecular specialist. He may find it necessary to lower your dosage level to below 1,000 milligrams daily. On the other hand, niacin's most common side effect—an uncomfortable, strong flushing of the skin—may be controlled by increasing the dose *slowly* over several weeks.

I probably take more vitamin supplements than my body actually requires. But I have found that these vitamins work well for me. If, perhaps, I waste a little money taking more supplements than I need, my recovery has certainly been worth the few extra dollars.

Our bodies give us many clues to which vitamins we need, but it is impossible for any of us to guess our particular nutritional requirements. The only way we can learn for sure what our optimal doses are is through blood-serum testing, which is the domain of the orthomolecular physician. Such things as water hardness, our choice of foods, soil conditions where the food is grown, shelf life and chemical contamination of the food, and our physical requirements due to stress and illness all make a difference in our body chemistry. If you do not know where to begin looking for an orthomolecular physician, contact the Princeton BioCenter, in Skillman, New Jersey (see Appendix A). The BioCenter does a comprehensive orthomolecular blood workup that uncovered the genetic link—pyroluria—causing the mental problems in my family for four generations.

If you are not currently taking vitamins or minerals and you plan to visit an orthomolecular physician or psychiatrist in the *near* future, do **not** begin taking any supplements now. Your physician will be able to get a clearer blood-chemistry picture of you. If you are currently taking vitamins or minerals, keep careful records so the doctor can analyze your test results accurately.

All of my nutrition books are fairly unanimous in their choice of vitamins, minerals, and other supplements for mentally disabled persons. In addition to niacin, it appears that zinc, manganese, magnesium, vitamin B-6, and vitamin B-12 may be especially important for Alzheimer's patients, 50 percent of whom, according to the Princeton BioCenter, lack these nutrients. A list of the vitamins and minerals that I take is in Table 3.1. I also take gingko biloba, an herbal remedy to improve memory that can be found in most health and natural-food stores, and watch my intake of protein. The Center for Disease Control, in Atlanta, reports that Alzheimer's victims do not have enough protein in their brains. Protein deficiency causes all sorts of mental dysfunctions. Dr. Huggins says that he has never seen a mercury-toxic dental patient recover after amalgam removal without eating animal protein. He recommends six ounces of red meat daily.

As far as what kind of supplements to take, multivitamin formulas are more likely to contain substances that brain-fogged people cannot tolerate, so purchase your vitamins separately. I use Bronson, Schiff, Mega Food, New Chapter, Rainbow Light, Perque, and Super Blue-Green Algae, to name a few. Perque vitamins seem well-named. I noticed a wonderful bounce of energy a few days after I started taking them. It happened again when my liquid potassium-mineral supplement finally kicked in after three or four weeks. I also like Super Blue-Green (freeze-dried) Algae. My friend's father, who had Alzheimer's disease, experienced a noticeable improvement, and I wouldn't be without it.

There are many fine vitamin and mineral supplements on the market. However, they are not cheap. It is expensive for supplement manufacturers to obtain pharmaceutical-grade materials, or to grow or purchase high-quality, organic fruits, vegetables, grains, and herbs for "natural" vitamins. Keeping fruits and vegetables fresh and capturing their energy without destroying enzymes or

Table 3.1. Vitamins and Minerals Generally Recommended for Mentally Disabled Persons

Nutrient	Major Uses	Comments
Vitamin A	Prevents night blindness and other eye problems. May be useful against acne and other skin disorders. Enhances immunity. May help prevent cancer. May heal gastrointestinal ulcers. Protects against pollution. Needed for epithelial-tissue maintenance and repair.	Mercury-toxic individuals must **not** get this vitamin from fish sources. Instead, they should get it from *beta-carotene*. The mega doses of vitamin A that cerebral allergy physicians recommend to brain-fogged patients can quickly build up and become toxic if fish sources are used. Excess vitamin A from beta-carotene sources, however, is excreted in the urine. In addition, if too much beta-carotene is eventually absorbed, you will know it immediately because your skin will turn the color of carrots.
B Complex B-1 (thiamin) B-2 (riboflavin) B-3 (niacin, niacinamide) B-6 (pyridoxine)	Maintains healthy nerves, skin, eyes, hair, liver, mouth, gastrointestinal-tract muscle tone. B vitamins are coenzymes involved in energy production. Emotional or physical stress increases need. May be useful against depression or anxiety.	Vitamin B-6 is involved in the synthesis and metabolism of many neurotransmitters and is, therefore, a factor in such mental afflictions as pyroluria (see Chapter 5). If you have difficulty remembering your dreams in the morning, you probably have a B-6 deficiency. The *pyridoxal 5 phosphate* (P5P) form of B-6 is five-to-ten times more effective than any other form.
B-12 (cobalamin)	Needed for fat and carbohydrate metabolism. Needed for prevention and treatment of B-12 anemia. Maintains proper nervous-system function. May be useful against anxiety and depression.	Hydroxycobalamin is the only form of this vitamin that Dr. Huggins recommends for mercury-toxic patients. The first indication of a B-12 deficiency, which causes pernicious anemia, will likely be psychosis. Caution: B-12 is stored in the body, so be careful you do not take too much.

Folic acid	Works closely with B-12. Involved in protein metabolism. Needed for healthy cell division and replication. Needed for prevention and treatment of folic acid anemia. Stress may increase need. May be useful against depression and anxiety. May be useful in treating cervical dysplasia. Oral contraceptives may increase need.	Folic acid is considered to be a brain food. Mercury blocks the function of folic acid in the body, and many of the symptoms of mercury toxicity are identical to those of folic-acid deficiency. Generally, vitamin B-12 must be taken in conjunction with folic acid, and vice versa, because if you take one without the other, you can cause a deficiency in the other.
Pantothenic acid	Needed in fat, protein, and carbohydrate metabolism. Needed for synthesis of hormones and cholesterol. Needed for red-blood-cell production. Needed for nerve transmission. Vital for healthy functioning of the adrenal glands. May be useful against joint inflammation. May be useful against depression and anxiety.	Pantothenic acid is known as the "antistress vitamin." Increased dosages are needed in times of stress. In addition, pantothenic acid is useful in combatting the symptoms of caffeine withdrawal.
Biotin	Needed for metabolism of protein,, fats, and carbohydrates. Not enough data available, but deficiencies may be implicated in high serum cholesterol, seborrheic dermatitis, and certain nervous-system disorders.	A deficiency of biotin may cause depression.

Choline	Involved in metabolism of fat and cholesterol, and absorption and utilization of fat. Makes an important brain neuro-transmitter.	Choline is necessary for proper nerve transmission. Without choline, brain function and memory become impaired.
Vitamin C (ascorbic acid)	Needed for growth and repair of tissues. May reduce cholesterol. Antioxidant. May help prevent cancer. Enhances immunity. Stress increases requirement. May reduce high blood pressure. May prevent atherosclerosis. Protects against pollution.	Cola addiction is a sign of vitamin C deficiency and can be reversed by drinking one teaspoon of powdered sodium ascorbate in a glass of water as soon as you wake up in the morning. Every time you crave another cola, take an additional quarter-teapoon in a glass of water. In three or four days, you will wonder why you ever liked cola drinks at all.
Vitamin D	Required for calcium and phosphorus absorption and utilization. Needed for prevention and treatment of osteoporosis. Enhances immunity.	Vitamin D is often deficient in the elderly. Be careful, however, because this is another vitamin that is stored in the body. You can accumulate too much of it, which may lead to atherosclerosis.
Vitamin K	Needed for blood clotting. May play a role in bone formation. May prevent osteoporosis.	Alzheimer's victims have a decrease of this vitamin in their hippocampus and cerebral cortex.[4] Caution: vitamin K is stored in the body.
Calcium	Needed for healthy bones and teeth. Needed for nerve transmission. Used for muscle function. May lower blood pressure. May prevent osteoporosis.	Mercury-toxic patients should not get this mineral from oyster sources because oyster shell may be contaminated with mercury. In addition, the calcium in many multivitamins may actually worsen a condition and contribute to "inactive" calcium being stored in the body. Use magnesium to balance it.

Magnesium	Needed for healthy bones. Involved in nerve transmission. Needed for muscle function. Used in energy formation. Needed for healthy blood vessels. May lower blood pressure.	A calcium-magnesium supplement, in addition to acting like a sedative, helps to eliminate underarm odors, which is especially helpful to Alzheimer's victims who suffer brain-fog reactions to underarm sprays containing aluminum.
Zinc	Needed for wound healing. Maintains taste and smell acuity. Needed for healthy immune system. Protects liver from chemical damage.	According to Dr. Jonathan Collin, an orthomolecular physician, "A zinc deficiency causes the intestine to malabsorb, which is an underlying cause of food allergies and many degenerative diseases." A zinc deficiency is indicated by white spots on the fingernails. When taking a zinc supplement, always take it in conjunction with vitamins B-6 and C. But be careful: zinc is stored in the body.
Iron	Vital for blood formation. Needed for energy production. Required for healthy immune system.	When taking iron, also take vitamin C, which can increase iron absorption by as much as 30 percent. But be careful: an iron excess has been found in association with Alzheimer's.
Copper	Involved in blood formation. Needed for healthy nerves. Needed for taste sensitivity. Used in energy production. Needed for healthy bone development.	Copper is a good mineral, but it can be stored in the brain, and many people with mental disorders have been found to have high levels there. In addition, chronic excessive exposure to copper is associated with an increased risk of dementia
Manganese	Needed for protein and fat metabolism. Used in energy formation.	Manganese acts as the key to unlocking the energy in a cell. The interruption of its metabolism is the greatest disturbance found in

| | Required for normal bone growth and reproduction. Needed for healthy nerves. Needed for healthy blood-sugar regulation. Needed for healthy immune system. | patients with such diseases as periodontal disease, arthritis, multiple sclerosis, muscular dystrophy, cancer, and heart disease. A deficiency in it is apt to be a primary one in all degenerative diseases. Tinnitus is often a symptom of deficiency. Mercury blocks its functioning. |
| Potassium | May lower blood pressure. Needed for energy storage. Needed for nerve transmission, muscle contraction, and hormone secretion. | If following a low-carbohydrate diet, be careful to get enough potassium. A lack of potassium can cause heart pain and arrhythmia, and lead to a heart attack. Take a slow-release potassium supplement, or get the mineral from parsley or the scrapings from the inside of banana peels. |

contaminating the product is a chemist's nightmare and a minor miracle. In addition, the manufacturers who really care about the quality of their products must compete financially with the low-end, diluted—what I call "junk"—vitamins and minerals on the shelves. You will get exactly what you pay for. If you want results, buy the premium brands found in health and natural-food stores.

I also take hydrochloric acid. You will need to take the Heidelberg Stomach Acid Test to determine your correct hydrochloric-acid dosage, or refer to Dr. Jonathan Wright's book *Healing With Nutrition*. In addition, I take two digestive enzymes ten to fifteen minutes before meals, two more about fifteen minutes after dinner, and two at bedtime. A calcium-magnesium combination seems to help me fall asleep at night and, I am delighted to say, eliminates underarm odors. (Many allergic people notice strong brain-fog reactions to underarm sprays, hair sprays—sprays of any sort.) And lately, I have also been taking a tablespoon of Spectrum Naturals Veg-Omega-3 fresh flax oil (expeller pressed) daily. My dry skin problems cleared up quickly, and I noticed increased energy.

For more information on nutritional supplements, there are many excellent books on the market. Four that I particularly liked are *Brainfood: Nutrition and Your Brain,* by Brian Morgan, M.D., and Roberta Morgan; *The Complete Guide to Your Emotions and Your Health: New Dimensions in Mind-Body Healing,* by Emrika Padus; and *Understanding Vitamins and Minerals* and *Fighting Disease,* both by the editors of *Prevention* magazine.

The sixth book on our must-read list is *Your Body Doesn't Lie,* by John Diamond, M.D. Be sure to read it before purchasing any vitamin or mineral supplement. While not totally up-to-date regarding brain allergies, this book will help you to pick out the vitamins, minerals, and foods that should cooperate best with your body. It might save you a lot of money. I threw away hundreds of dollars worth of products that caused me severe brain-fog reactions before reading it.

Voll testing is also a quick and easy—and probably more accurate—method for assuring biocompatibility. In addition, a little-known book entitled *Which Vitamins and Herbs Do I Need?,* from the Biokinesiology Institute, gives a supposedly even more accurate testing method for identifying the most beneficial supplements for you.

The seventh book on the must-read list is *Feed Yourself Right,* by Lendon Smith, M.D. Pay particular attention to the discussion of vitamin injections. If you are deficient in nutrients, your body will not be able to absorb vitamins through your intestines. The intramuscular B-complex vitamins recommended by Dr. Smith are available over-the-counter in Canadian and Mexican pharmacies. Intramuscular folic acid, however, requires a prescription from your physician.

Danger: Do not attempt to give yourself injections without the proper instruction. You could paralyze yourself by inserting the needle in the wrong site. Have a nurse show your spouse or other helper how to combine the three recommended vitamins into one 3-cc., 23-gauge syringe (one shot hurts less) and how to administer the shot in your buttocks. The rubber top on the Canadian vitamin container might dull the needle, which you'll have to replace, but otherwise, the shot is nearly painless if the needle is inserted quickly and the contents administered over a period of two to three minutes.

Two other books that I have found very useful are *Let's Get Well*, by Adelle Davis, and *How to Get Well*, by Paavo Airola. I usually check Dr. Smith's book against Adelle Davis's book, and take the less traumatic, and less expensive, action.

STRESS, EMOTIONS, AND ALLERGIES

Allergies are like a barrel of water. They are not bothersome until the barrel is full and they start spilling over the side. Do whatever is necessary to reduce the stress in your daily life. Your attitude will have a lot to do with your recovery. Concentrate on the good things in your life. Read *The Complete Guide to Your Emotions and Your Health: New Dimensions in Mind-Body Healing*, by Emrika Padus and the editors of *Prevention* magazine.

Sometimes, people defer seeking happiness at the best possible time and place: the here and now. The pursuit of positive future goals is good, but the too-avid pursuit of anything is not. Concentrating solely on the future can rob you of the happiness available today. "Keeping busy" can be an acceptable way subconsciously and socially to avoid facing a difficult issue. But it can also be unhealthy. You need to take some time out to smell the flowers. Take some time out to think. If you could do anything right now, what would you choose?

If Alzheimer's or another disease have turned you into a couch potato with a television remote-control stuck to your hand, get up off your duff. There are very few diseases that a daily three-mile walk or one-mile swim will not quickly nudge into remission. Get out! Go have some active fun—preferably with someone you care for. I walk approximately five miles, three times a week, through a beautiful park near the sea.

If you are not actively seeking a healthy lifestyle and relationship, or if you are ignoring any present health risks or medical problems, ask yourself these questions: Am I afraid to face life? Do I really want to live? Or would I rather die? Take time to think carefully about your answers. They might surprise you.

Making a new friend is giving yourself a present. When I reflect upon my life, I regret that I desired *things* more than *friends*. There came a time when I began to acquire everything I thought I wanted. But I was miserable, and I became ill and lost everything anyway. Things are just things—a poor substitute for friends.

I do not intend to waste whatever time I have remaining. I am recovered now, and it is time for me to begin taking new risks—to face new challenges and start enjoying life again. I promised myself decades ago to walk the Pacific Coast Trail, which stretches from Mexico to Canada; I have an eagle, a fox, and a thrush to visit. There is a bear cub I once photographed and promised to greet again. He should be very old by now. I wonder if he is still alive. A tiller, full sheets before the wind, and mounting rolling seas beckon. These years of sickness have taken their toll on my spirit, and I am now as stale as moldy hardtack. I yearn for new adventures.

Allergies are gaining more and more attention nowadays as the world is becoming more polluted. Doctors in general are becoming more aware of the role that allergies play in diseases. If you have any allergies, take care of them. This chapter gave you a brief overview of how. And if you are experiencing any severe allergic reactions, especially burning-brain sensations, find a clinical ecologist immediately.

In Chapter 4, we will discuss the third leg of the milking stool: diet and nutrition.

4.

You Are What You Eat

*The best doctors in the world are Doctor Diet,
Doctor Quiet, and Doctor Merryman.*

—Jonathan Swift
English satirist

At first blush, it would seem to be a tragedy that so many allergies arise because of food and eating. Eating is an activity so many enjoy, and food is supposedly our life-blood. But on the other hand, when we carefully analyze how far today's society has strayed from the diet nature meant the human body to ingest, maybe it's not so hard to understand.

When he was the Surgeon General of the United States, Dr. C. Everett Koop reported that if we do not smoke or drink excessively, our diet can influence our long-term health prospects more than anything else we do. To look at his statement in another way, nearly all the cells in our body are eventually replaced with brand-new cells.

The vitality of these new cells depends on the quality of the foods we eat.

Compare tired, ailing cells to the dirt and grease in dishwater. The body constantly cleanses itself by sloughing off toxins and these ailing, aging, tired cells the same way we drain dirty, greasy water from a sink. Proper nutrition and vitamin supplementation can be compared to fresh, pristine water. Run fresh water into the sink and watch the filthy water turn clear again.

After a long, hard winter, deer instinctively eat the tips of new growth. These buds give them vitality and sleek new fur. Why should people be any different? There are *dead* foods, which are highly processed, packaged foods, and *live* foods, which have energy and life stored within them, such as fresh vegetables and fruits.

Milk and wheat are near the top of the list of foods to which most allergy patients react. But there are many others. Sugar, for instance, is not far down the list.[1] There are also some allergy-producing substances that are not a food themselves but are linked with food, e.g., chemicals such as food coloring and insecticides.

Based on Dr. Huggins' remarks in *It's All in Your Head,* as well as on the low-carbohydrate diet that Dr. Richard Kunin recommends in his book *Mega-Nutrition: The New Prescription for Maximum Health, Energy and Longevity,* I would hesitate to suggest avoiding meat protein completely, at least until the mercury has been released from your body. However, be very careful about where your meat comes from, and use meat as a side dish rather than the main part of your meals. If possible, *never eat fat*; the fat layer is where the body sends the pollution it cannot dispose of quickly enough through the kidneys. Additionally, researchers at the Nathan Pritikin Research Foundation have found that it takes six months to induce adult-onset diabetes in a healthy individual through the ingestion of excessive amounts of sugar, but only six weeks through the ingestion of excessive amounts of fats.

Celiac disease can be another problem. Food allergies in general—and in particular to the gluten protein found in wheat, rye, barley, oats, and buckwheat—cause celiac disease. Celiac disease, in turn, causes malabsorption, which can cause the brain to starve to death. Furthermore, Dr. Chris Reading, co-author of *Your Family Tree Connection,* links schizophrenia, Alzheimer's, multiple sclerosis, thyroid disorders, pernicious anemia, lymphomas, bowel cancers, leukemia, arthritis, and diabetes with food allergies and nutritional deficiencies.

What can we do to combat the effects of food allergies? That's what we'll look at in this chapter.

ALLERGY TESTING

Unfortunately, there is no scratch or blood test available today that is reliable enough to identify *every* substance that provokes a cerebral brain-fog reaction. But such a test is exactly what schizophrenics and Alzheimer's sufferers need. The faster and more accurately the specific chemicals, foods, pollens, and other substances causing brain fog can be identified and eliminated, the better the potential for recovery.

I expect that because of this, provocative testing will remain necessary in brain-fog cases. Provocative testing thoroughly isolates each suspected substance. But the one-on-one nature of the testing procedure is time consuming and necessarily expensive, and the reactions are occasionally intense. For example, a lovely young woman I knew suffered an acute convulsive reaction for five hours after eating three cherries. In another example, a violent prisoner I read about exhibited unpredictable behavior that authorities were unable to understand or control. The prisoner was provocatively tested for one of his favorite foods—eggs—and immediately became explosively violent. A half-dozen guards were required to overpower him, even though he was tightly bound in a straitjacket. Needless to say, the man doesn't eat eggs anymore.

In August 1990, *The New England Journal of Medicine* published a seven-year-old study based on a test that one of my clinical ecologists, Dr. David Buscher, refused to participate in because he felt the protocol was flawed. The report indicated that provocative allergy testing is inaccurate. Based on my experience, I believe this is wrong. No other allergy test available is more accurate at uncovering substances causing brain fog or works better to teach a patient how to protect himself. I say this after having had every allergy test there is.

The real issue, I believe, is economics. I strongly feel that clinical ecologists are taking too much business away from traditional allergists, who do scratch testing, and that traditional allergists are just protecting their turf. Scratch testing *for cerebral allergies,* I have found, is a waste of money and time. Traditional allergists, however, are not trained in clinical ecology, nor are they able to duplicate clinical ecology results.

Before we move on, let me stress that you should never test yourself. And never eat any foods you might be allergic to on an empty stomach. Your reaction in either case could be cataclysmic. I am terribly allergic to both milk and wheat. On one occasion, I foolishly tested them both, at home, at the same time, after having fasted for five days. My cerebral reaction was so severe that I felt compelled to stop it at all costs—even the ultimate one. In addition, do not consider provocative testing anywhere if you have any heart irregularities. But if you do decide to get tested, the doctor's office is the place to do it. Clinical ecologists know how to interrupt severe reactions and handle any emergencies.

For more information on the allergy tests available today, and for referrals to clinical ecologists, please see Appendices A and B.

NUTRITION AND THE LOW-CARBOHYDRATE DIET

The eighth book you should read is *Mega-Nutrition: The New Prescription for Maximum Health, Energy and Longevity*, by Richard Kunin, M.D., paying special attention to his low-carbohydrate diet, and nutrition and vitamin suggestions. Be careful, though: don't carry a good plan to extremes. Completely eliminating carbohydrates from your diet is dangerous. In fact, do not cut your carbohydrate intake to below 40 grams of complex carbohydrates daily, then work back to 60 grams within two weeks. Reducing carbohydrates to below 60 grams can have dangerous side effects, even though you feel better after the first week of dieting. Depletion of potassium can cause heart pain, which may be indicative of an impending heart attack. This can be remedied by taking slow-release potassium, available by prescription, or by eating parsley or the scrapings from the inside of banana peels. In addition, eating too much protein without adequate carbohydrate intake will eventually leach calcium and protein, and over time, cause painful gall and kidney stones to form.

Also vital for low-carbohydrate dieters are nutritional supplements. Water rapidly leaches the water-soluble vitamins and minerals, along with salt, from the body. Regular vitamin, mineral, and salt supplementation is *absolutely necessary* to provide the brain with additional nutritional support on a low-carbohydrate diet.

Watch how you cheat on a low-carbohydrate diet. I was hooked on cola drinks as much as any addict, and was morbidly obese and feeling generally miserable. My physician said my whole family had diabetes, and he put me on a low-carbohydrate diet and Phenformin, which is a discontinued diabetes medication. Over the next thirty days, I hand-thatched two-thirds of an acre of lawn, planted twenty rhododendrons, sold a ton of insurance, and lost forty pounds. I was literally bouncing with new-found energy. But when I went off the regimen, I courted disaster.

My wife makes the finest apple pie I have ever tasted. Occasionally, she would make one for herself (I was not supposed to have any), and over a period of a week or so, taking a sliver here and there, she would slowly consume it. One time, she left a very small piece—the last of the pie—in the refrigerator, and I—on the low-carbohydrate-diet wagon for thirty days—made a bad decision: I ate that slice of pie, plus a package of soda crackers and a big glass of milk. In twenty minutes, my mind was as zonked as if I had slugged down six Singapore slings and a rum chaser. As if that wasn't enough, my body felt ancient and battered.

Arguing against low-carbohydrate diets are Dr. Chris Reading and Ross Meillon, authors of *Your Family Tree Connection*, who say that such a diet can cause schizophrenia. I, however, strongly feel it does not, provided there is adequate vitamin and mineral supplementation, the 60-gram level for carbohydrates is maintained, and the carbohydrates consumed come from a variety of fresh vegetables and brown rice instead of junk food. Read both books carefully and decide for yourself what you think.

Dr. William G. Crook, who wrote *The Yeast Connection* and *The Yeast Connection Cookbook*, says, "The reason low-carbohydrate diets work is simply this: Such diets avoid common foods people are sensitive to, including yeast, wheat, corn and other foods, as well as sugar." Dr. Crook believes a high-complex-carbohydrate diet is preferable to a low-carbohydrate diet.

Diet is certainly an important facet of controlling food allergies causing brain fog. I address three separate diets in this book. In theory, the perfect diet, I believe, is the high-complex-carbohydrate diet that Dr. Crook suggests combined with the four-day rotation diet that Dr. Theron Randolph recommends (see page 91). In practice, however, people with too many cerebral allergies cannot think clearly enough to either cook for themselves or follow any program without extraordinary discipline. But it is possible for them to stick with a low-carbohydrate diet until their thought process clears enough to be able to participate in the other programs.

If you opt for a low-carbohydrate diet, I suggest you join Overeaters Anonymous (see Appendix C). Overeaters Anonymous has used the low-carbohydrate diet successfully for more than fifteen years *without* any side effects. Members will stand up at their meetings and tell everyone that sugar, white flour, and junk foods are poison with the same fervor as Temperance League women breaking up a saloon before Prohibition. As a matter of fact, this was nearly how my own physician acted. He was adamant about fighting diabetes and insisted I start a low-carbohydrate diet. He was, I thought, a smart G.P. whose practice included psychiatry and geriatrics. I just wish he had also realized the need for vitamin and mineral supplementation.

NUTRITION AND CANCER

If you have any type of cancer or diabetes, please read *The McDougall Plan*, by John A. McDougall, M.D., and

Mary A. McDougall. John McDougall is a practicing physician who uses a dietary approach to treating disease, and his wife, Mary, is a nurse who specializes in nutrition. Together, they wrote this book that explodes the dietary myths of Western civilization.

Just looking at their chapter titles gives you a rough idea of their program: "Red Meat, Poultry, and Fish are Avoided on a Health-Supporting Diet," "Dairy Products and Eggs are Avoided on a Health-Supporting Diet," and "A Health-Supporting Diet Contains No Cholesterol." Other things they feel a healthy diet should avoid include fats, too much protein, unprotected simple sugars, and food additives, including salt. Instead, they stress the importance of complex carbohydrates.

The McDougall diet is a true vegetarian diet, not a lacto-ovo-vegetarian plan. In addition, it is not a diet in the sense that most people think of a diet, but rather, a life-long change in eating habits. Nathan Pritikin, in the "Foreword" to the book, says, "This program is strict, and those who wish to follow it must be motivated to make a complete break with their life-long food habits." He adds that it "establishes vegetarianism as a healthful way of life based on the latest scientific data and should give comfort to those considering making this dietary change."

Another good book for diabetics and cancer victims is *Nutrition: The Cancer Answer,* by Maureen Salaman.

WHOLESOME FOODS

Senior citizens should purchase the freshest, most wholesome foods available. Europeans use small refrigerators because they buy their food fresh nearly every day. I have a friend whose father, in his eighties, recovered from senility by getting off the local senior-citizen meal-delivery program and buying his own fresh vegetables.

If you park your teeth in a glass of water at night, it is very likely that you do not chew your food well enough. Some of the larger food particles may pass through your intestinal wall and, not recognized as nutrition by your body, will be attacked as foreign invaders, causing many food allergies. Food processors can help solve this problem.

George Roni, at ninety-three years of age, threw away his glasses, which he had needed for reading for many years, because he changed his dietary habits after his wife died. He began purchasing the highest quality meats available, which he cuts into small cubes, combines with many fresh vegetables from his garden and a few whole grains, and tosses into a pot on the stove. Good eating does not have to be complicated or expensive.

THE FOUR-DAY FOOD-ROTATION DIET

One of my allergists said, "The Greeks knew more than two thousand years ago that people who did not eat a particular food, in any form, more often than every four days were healthier, stronger, and felt very well." Today's allergists agree.

For many years, clinical ecologists have been recommending food rotation diets to all allergy patients, regardless of their medical complaints. This type of diet has been responsible for curing many patients of diverse chronic diseases. Then, Dr. Theron Randolph discovered the environmental-pollution—health connection. When a patient combines a food rotation diet with the avoidance of chemical contaminants in his food and environment, he improves remarkably.

Most nutrition books recommend growing a home garden to avoid chemical contamination of produce and to get peak vitamin and mineral content. If I understand correctly, the average shelf life of vegetables in the market is two months. If you cannot grow your own vegetables, try to wash off as many pesticides from your store-bought produce as possible. Cut the top half-inch off apples. Be careful where you shop: some chemically sensitive cerebral-allergy patients have passed out in the vegetable departments of supermarkets. It is hard to believe but the average person in the United States consumes approximately seven pounds of chemicals every year.

Organically grown fruits and vegetables, as well as more processed foods, can be found in natural-food stores. Be sure to look for "certified organic" labeling. Also, in local farmers' markets, you can find organic growers, many of whom have been growing organically for a number of years, using natural pesticides and fertilizers as opposed to the chemical varieties.

I have found that when I completely avoid sugar, flour, milk, coffee, soda pop, fruit juice, canned and packaged foods, monosodium glutamate (MSG), and food coloring, and take my digestive enzymes, stomach acid, vitamins, and minerals—plus walk regularly and stay away from chemical pollution—I feel twenty-five years younger and think very clearly.

Another book by Adelle Davis, *You Can Get Well*, includes calorie, vitamin, and mineral charts for 287 foods. You should find these charts very helpful.

EXERCISE

Whatever else you do, you need to undertake a regular, moderate exercise program or you will never completely recover.[2] I know a woman who, at one time, could only walk a hundred feet at a clip but now walks seven miles a day. Her husband, a physician, closes his office at lunchtime and walks with her. They repeat their stroll in the evening.

No matter how depressed, grouchy, or tired you are, make yourself walk. Moderate exercise is an excellent way to clear away low feelings and brain fog. Depression and brain fog will always lift if you walk far enough. One of my physicians told me not to worry about finding my way back home. If I walked far enough, she said, my head would clear and I would regain my strength. She was correct.

Many years ago, when I was at my worst and could not stand my suffering anymore, I planned to commit suicide. I was terribly confused, depressed, and out of shape. Fortunately, I decided to walk to a remote area. Several hours later, when I arrived there, I laid down on the grass to rest. I looked at the thousands of breathtaking stars in the sky and realized my brain fog had lifted—and that I felt much better. I thought, "You dummy, go on home." After that, I walked every night, which saved my life. My family immediately noticed that I became more easygoing. And best of all, my confusion departed.

Walk at 3:00 A.M. if necessary. But do not walk near vehicle exhaust fumes. If you don't do anything else I recommend in this book, promise yourself one thing: never commit suicide until you have walked ten miles. A word to the wise: bring a quarter for the telephone.

PSYCHOTROPIC MEDICATIONS

Falling under the heading of "diet and nutrition" are medications. Although most people do not look at them as nutrients, they are ingested and are considered to be a food.

Most medications do not cause a problem. Some do. Some are fine for the average person but can be dangerous

for an Alzheimer's sufferer. Every psychiatrist in the
United States is trained to control bizarre behavior with
psychotropic medications even though, so often, the side
effects of these medications can be devastating. The patient may lose every behavioral attribute that we call
human. There are alternatives to psychotropic medications, however—alternatives that are more effective and
do not have side effects. All the medical specialties we
discuss in this book are an example. But one medical
specialty shines above the rest: homeopathy. Homeopathic physicians seem to be able to correct all sorts of
behavior, mood, and thought problems, and with *no bad
side effects*. I once knew a mental-health professional
whose personality was so easygoing, it was almost flat.
She was taking 200 milligrams of the psychotropic medication Sinequan every day. She finally visited a homeopathic physician, plus had all her silver-amalgam fillings
replaced, and was eventually able to reduce her medication to 50 milligrams of Sinequan every other day. Today,
she is off medications completely.

At least seven psychotropic medications that cause
problems are referred to in the pharmaceutical references
Facts and Comparisons and *Physicians' Desk Reference*. These medications, which are also known as
"phenothiazines," can cause cerebral edema (swelling), according to the reference books. These drugs are listed in
Table 4.1.

Dr. Randolph found that patients who were taking any
psychotropic medications for an extended period of time
did not do well in his environmental hospital unit. Clinical
ecology hospital treatment is designed to last for only
about twenty-four days, and it takes six *weeks* to "dry out"
from psychotropic drugs. If you have been taking a psychotropic medication, see an orthomolecular physician or

Table 4.1. Psychotropic Medications That
May Cause Cerebral Swelling

Generic Name	Trade Name
Chlorpromazine	Thorazine
Promazine	Sparine
Triflupromazine	Vesprin
Thioridazine	Mellaril
Medoridazine	Serentil
Perphenazine	Trilafon
Prochlorperazine	Compazine

psychiatrist first. Wait to see a clinical ecologist until you
are clean.

Psychotropic medications are not the only trou-
blemakers, however. The AARP warns senior citizens to
beware of more common prescription and over-the-counter drugs, too, since many may produce symptoms that
mimic senile dementia. Some of the medications that can
do this are tranquilizers, pain relievers, eyedrops, adrenal
steroids, certain gastrointestinal medications, glaucoma
drugs, blood-pressure medications, and digitalis. The
grandmother of one of my friends was diagnosed as having
Alzheimer's, but it was eventually discovered that she was
instead having brain-fog reactions to her medications.

Older patients should not accept prescription-drug-in-
duced problems as being part of the normal aging process.
They are not. Luckily, however, the AARP says, "Often
when these drugs are stopped, the condition disappears."

A PHARMACIST'S STORY

No symptom should just be accepted as a part of growing
old. Every symptom has a reason for being. The following
story illustrates my point.

The woman looked bewildered. She asked her husband, "Is it snowing outside?" "How did I get here?" "Did I just come in?" Her husband suspected a stroke and telephoned their family doctor immediately.

Before going to work, the woman had had an appointment with the doctor. The physician had given her a new prescription: indomethacin for phlebitis.

The woman is a responsible pharmacist. Not one person in the pharmacy had suspected anything was amiss. She had taken the medication shortly before leaving the store. She knows drug interactions and side effects. She was, at the time, forty-five years old and in relatively good health. She drove twenty-four miles—difficult miles through a snowstorm—to get home, but once home, she was unaware that she had driven or how she had gotten there. The whole evening, in fact, was erased from her memory.

This story may be dramatic, but it is not bizarre. Prescription-drug reactions can sneak up so slowly that they go unnoticed and become masked as other symptoms. There is a reason for every symptom. There is a reason for memory problems. Do not just pass anything over as old age.

MAKING MEDICATIONS SAFER

Responsible consumerism extends into the area of taking medications. Do not just accept every drug for which your doctor gives you a prescription, or that he advises you to buy over-the-counter, without asking questions. A truly wise pharmaceutical consumer will observe the following precautions:

• Dump *all* your medications into a sack and take them to your primary doctor. Review every medication: the need for taking it, its dosage, its frequency, how long you should take it, and its possible side effects. Find out if you can stop taking any of them. Discuss any possible interactions between those you must continue.

- Make sure that either you or a friend understands exactly how you should be taking each medication. *Ask your pharmacist.*
- Assume that any symptom you develop after starting a new medication is a drug reaction. *Report it to your physician immediately.*
- Every time you add a new medication, see if you can drop an old one.
- If a specialist gives you a new prescription, check it with your primary doctor first.
- Do not use generic substitutes. They may not be identical to what the doctor prescribed, and may not produce the same effects.
- Don't jump around among several different pharmacies. And stay away from mail-order prescription services. Your regular, hometown pharmacist knows you best and is more likely to catch any subtle changes in your health that may require further investigation or an alteration in your medications. Your pharmacist is a good person to know on a first-name basis.
- Don't ask your doctor for a pill you can do without.
- Play it safe. Do not interrupt or talk with a pharmacist when he, or she, is filling a prescription. Concentration is required to avoid making a mistake. Wait until the pharmacist can give you his full attention.
- If you are on diuretics, high-blood-pressure or heart medication, or a low-carbohydrate diet *and have memory problems*, ask your physician to check your electrolytes. Electrolytes conduct the body's electricity through the system, and when they are all working correctly, the body is said to be in electrolytic balance.

People on the aforementioned medications or diet, however, tend to expel a lot of water, which can disrupt the electrolytic balance. Once the balance is out of whack, it is often difficult to restore, and the sufferer's health may quickly deteriorate. A heart attack may be one result. Therefore, it is important to have your electrolytes checked when you note a concern.

• Dump all your discontinued medications down the toilet. Keep them out of the reach of youngsters.

Medications are supposed to help, not hurt. But it takes a wise consumer to keep this so. Be an active consumer and you'll be a winning consumer.

These, then, are the three legs of the milking stool: amalgam removal, allergy care, and proper nutrition. They are three legs that should pick you up off the floor and support you very sturdily. However, this three-legged milking stool, as I have said, works not only for Alzheimer's victims, but also for the sufferers of many other afflictions, most notably schizophrenia. Before closing this book, therefore, let's take a closer look—in Chapter 5—at that also-misunderstood illness.

5.

The Other Side of the Coin: Schizophrenia

The trouble with people is not that [they] don't know but that they know so much that ain't so.

—Henry Wheeler Shaw
("Josh Billings")
American humorist

I have been personally involved with the psychiatric community, for one reason or another, for more than fifty years. I have watched psychiatrists apply nearly every modality of treatment conceivable to the hapless patients who fall into their institutional-caretaker hands—from straitjackets, beatings, padded cells, football helmets, electric shock treatments, and lobotomies; through the talk therapies; to the present psychotropic medications; and back to electric shock again. I have two observations regarding traditional schizophrenia therapies. First, not one of them works! Each of the above treatment processes is an attempt to mask symptoms or to modify and control behavior. Not one permanently cures schizophrenia.

Second, since the psychiatric community has not found the cure for schizophrenia, it is time to recognize that schizophrenia is a medical, not a psychiatric, ailment and to listen to other medical specialists who may have a better handle on curing it. If psychiatrists continue to restrict themselves to considering and utilizing information exclusively from within their own field, they may never be able to cure schizophrenia, any more than neurologists have been able to cure Alzheimer's disease.

I strongly believe that schizophrenia is the other side of the coin to Alzheimer's. It may even be the same side of the coin, a sister illness sharing the same parents, or at least a half-sister with one parent the same. In this chapter, I'd like to present my personal findings about this mysterious affliction that strikes about 8 percent of Americans every year, according to the Alzheimer's and Related Disorders Association, based in Chicago. If part of the roots are the same, I believe that at least part of the cure should be, too.

THE IMMUNE RESPONSE

It is not enough to be exposed to germs to come down with a disease. Every family doctor, nurse, and pharmacist knows that the body has to first be in a weakened condition. It must be an acceptable host.

The nuns on Molokai, in the Hawaiian Islands, are an example. They have been taking care of leprosy patients for more than eighty years now, but not one has ever contracted the disease herself. At the first sign of even a cold, a nun is transferred off the island.

Another example concerns a medical missionary at a remote African hospital who worked with hundreds of patients with communicable diseases. The missionary's colleagues feared for his life, until he took a disease culture and placed it directly on his skin to prove their fears were groundless. His friends, using a microscope, watched the germs die.

Perhaps the most dramatic example involves Louis Pasteur, who developed the pasteurization process, and Antoine Bechamp, his nineteenth-century contemporary and adversary over this germ idea. Professor Bechamp held a container in his hand full of enough bacteria to kill a dozen men. Pasteur told him that if he was so sure that germs cannot make a healthy person sick, he should drink the toxins. Bechamp, thereupon, turned to his assistant and told him to drink the bacteria. The man suffered no ill effects.

Compare your immune system to a receptacle. If you reside in the country, living close to the soil and eating fresh, natural foods, you might have an immune system that could be compared to a huge wine vat. But Americans left their farms after 1945. If your parents did this, and you have spent your life eating packaged, highly processed (dead) foods, your immune system might be compared to a rain barrel. If you have chronic disease in your lineage, the way I do, your immune system might be compared to a bucket.

Now think of bacteria, formaldehyde, mercury, hydrocarbons, toxins, and chemicals, along with neuroses, financial woes, job problems, marital difficulties, modern lifestyles . . . the list is endless. These are stressors. Now dump these stressors, one by one, into the wine vat, barrel, or bucket, and watch the water level rise. You cannot get a disease until the water reaches the top of the receptacle and the first drop spills over. As soon as that first drop of water dribbles over the rim and down the side, you have passed your immune threshold. Can you see the plus of having a wine vat instead of a bucket?

What direction your immune dysfunction takes depends on your heredity. It's like jumping out of an airplane without a parachute. Whether you land on Alzheimer's, schizophrenia, multiple sclerosis, cancer, or another disease, or just have to pay your doctor sixty dollars for a prescription to help you through the flu, depends on your immune system's weakest link or the virus to which it was exposed.

THE BODY-MIND CONNECTION

The body and mind may be so inexorably intertwined that it might be nearly impossible to separate emotional disorders from physical allergy responses. Based on what I have been able to determine from my research, I believe the mixed-up thought processes that characterize schizophrenia are not caused nearly so much by psychological maladaptive responses to life situations as to cerebral allergies due to environmental contamination, digestive disorders, malnutrition, and other metabolic disorders.

Professor Ronald Glaser, a virologist with the Ohio State University College of Medicine, supports my belief. He was quoted by Steven Findlay and Shannon Browniee in "The Delicate Dance of the Body and Mind," a short article in the July 2, 1990, issue of *U.S. News and World Report*. In the article, he says, "It is convenient to think of the body and mind as separate, but they are clearly not, and eventually, that has to change the whole of medicine."

Also supporting my belief are the scientists at the National Institute of Mental Health, according to an article, "Brave New World," by Nancy C. Anderson, M.D., published in the January 1990 issue of *Vogue* magazine. The scientists, according to Dr. Anderson, found shrunken[1] or abnormally developed brain tissue in fifteen sets of identical twins. Among these twins, they found that the

regions of the brain responsible for memory, emotion, and decision making were smaller in the schizophrenics.

In addition, Dr. Anderson, writing in the same article, says that magnetic resonance imaging (MRI) and CAT scans have revealed that "some patients with schizophrenia have enlarged, fluid filled cavities inside the brain as well as an excess of the external fluid that cushions the brain. The increased fluid may be the result of a loss of brain tissue possibly due to injury, drug use, poor maternal nutrition, etc. Similar tissue loss is seen in Alzheimer's, alcoholism, anorexia nervosa and bulimia." She adds, "If the alcoholic stops drinking and the anorexic or bulimic person returns to normal weight, the shrinkage is reversed."

John T. A. Ely, Ph.D., a biochemistry researcher, cites another body-mind connection in his article, "More on the Question of Neurotoxicity Due to Mercury in Dental Amalgams." He says that urine porphyrin is elevated when mercury toxicity is the principle predisposing factor in Alzheimer's, anorexia nervosa, multiple sclerosis, and Parkinson's, among other diseases. He also says mercury is indirectly involved with aysautonomias and autoimmune diseases, due to enzyme poisoning, and with Campylobacter pyloritis colonization and yeast overgrowth, which are believed to result in symptoms such as multiple hypersensitivities to foods, decreased T-cell function, and premenstrual syndrome.

Dr. Russell Jaffe, the director of the Princeton Bio-Center, agrees. He says schizophrenia and Alzheimer's disease may be related to toxic metals and adverse reactions to chemicals. After reviewing my material, he wrote, in a letter to me, "Your information about the role of cerebral allergy in Alzheimer's Syndrome is a well presented, well grounded exposition of the important relationship, often

overlooked, between cerebral late-phase immune responses ('delayed allergy') and the Alzheimer's condition." Everything that I have learned about Alzheimer's
and schizophrenia, and every action that I took to reverse
them in me, supports his observation.

And the connections continue. To repeat an example I
used in Chapter 1, Shannon Browniee, in her article,
"The Body at War: Baring the Secrets of the Immune
System," says, "More lethal still is the poisonous surfeit of
hormones produced by the overreacting immune system.
These hormones, called lymphokines, make mischief in
surrounding tissue and organs, causing swelling [cerebral
allergic response] and fever. . . . The effect of superantigens is so murderously swift. . . ."

Another article, "Aspirin May Help Prevent Alzheimer's," published in the May 7, 1990, issue of the *Skagit
Valley Herald*, reports, "A study by neuroscientist Pat
McGeer, M.D., Ph.D., and his wife, [organic chemist]
Edith McGeer, Ph.D., suggests anti-inflammatory drugs,
such as ASA tablets like aspirin, may prevent the development of Alzheimer's. Alzheimer's disease is rare among
rheumatoid arthritis patients, who take anti-inflammatory
drugs regularly to relieve joint swelling and stiffness."
From all reports, however, aspirin is probably too toxic for
Alzheimer's victims. Dristan, or some other anti-inflammatory medication safer than aspirin and not containing
aluminum, would be a better choice.

And a final body-mind connection: DNA technology
has revealed a genetic pattern of heredity in multiple
sclerosis and rheumatoid arthritis. Many researchers suspect an inherited defect will be found underlying all such
illnesses.[2] I believe that malformed genes, as well as the
plaque and tangles found in the brains of Alzheimer's
patients, are the end result—not the root cause—of Alzheimer's disease. Furthermore, I believe that endogenous

depression, schizophrenia, and Alzheimer's disease—as well as many other brain abnormalities, possibly including amyotrophic lateral sclerosis (ALS), Parkinson's disease, and multiple sclerosis—are intertwined and reversible. If either parent has a damaged chromosome, that gene may be passed on to his or her children. According to Dr. Huggins, "Studies have shown that the red blood cells (good mercury carriers) of the unborn infant contain 30 percent more mercury than the mother's."

This does not necessarily mean that schizophrenia and Alzheimer's are inevitable or irreversible. It does mean, however, that the children of sufferers need to live the most wholesome, environmentally uncontaminated lifestyle possible. It also means that neither psychotherapy nor psychotropic medications are an effective treatment for schizophrenia. The first is an expensive waste of time. The second usually has too many side effects.

Again, I speak not only from my research but also from my personal experience. I once met a woman who was obsessed with the thought that her husband was having an affair. (He was not.) Much to her psychologist's credit, he suspected her distress was caused by an underlying allergic response and referred her to a clinical ecologist. When I met the woman, I told her that every morning, I used to wake up feeling great and glad to be alive, but five minutes after I showered, sprayed my underarms with a deodorant, and used my wife's hairspray, I became a mean, explosive jerk. It always seemed to me that my wife or daughter was at fault when, in fact, it was me, or rather, the inability of my liver and immune system to metabolize the chlorine and other chemicals to which I had exposed myself. A surprised look registered on the woman's face. She recognized that the only time she experienced her hallucinations was in the shower. The solution was simple. She purchased whole-house and point-of-use water filters.

OBSCURE METABOLIC DISORDERS
CAUSING SCHIZOPHRENIA

Over the years, as the research into schizophrenia—and Alzheimer's—picks up speed in the right direction, I believe many obscure causes will be uncovered. I feel that most of the causes will fall into the areas we just discussed in this book: metal toxicity, allergy, and nutritional deficiency. The following little-known metabolic disorders, I am certain, will be fair examples.

Celiac Disease

Celiac disease, which is a gluten-induced disease of the intestinal tract, is probably the *leading* overlooked cause of psychosis. Induced by an allergy to gluten—which is found in wheat, rye, barley, oats, and buckwheat—it involves atrophy in the intestines, which results in a loss of absorptive surface area. Nutrients, including especially vitamin B-12 and folic acid, are therefore malabsorbed.

When psychosis and celiac disease are both present, the malnutrition caused by celiac disease most likely prevented the brain from protecting itself against methyl mercury and other environmental pollutants. The cure is simple: allergy testing and a gluten-free diet.

Pyroluria

Dr. Chris Reading, in *Your Family Tree Connection*, says that he believes at least 30 percent of the people admitted with schizophrenia to Australia's mental hospitals have pyroluria. The Princeton BioCenter reports the figure to be 42 percent of all psychiatric patients worldwide.

Pyroluria is a familial disorder frequently characterized by low serum immune globulin A (IgA). It is a stress-induced disorder that results in a deficiency of vitamin B-6 and zinc. Pyroluria is marked by a high level of pyrroles in the urine. Pyrroles are organic compounds that combine first with B-6 and then with zinc. They are excreted via the urine, taking the B-6 and zinc with them and causing the double deficiency. Other symptoms of the disorder include an inability to remember dreams, morning nausea, an inability to eat breakfast, nervous exhaustion, severe inner tension, a fear of people, sore joints, insomnia, and distorted perception.

Pyroluria is the easiest of all mental afflictions to cure. Testing the urine identifies the problem, which is then easily corrected with B-6 and zinc supplementation. The test should be a part of the admission procedure to all mental hospitals.

If you feel you might have pyroluria, contact the Princeton BioCenter (see Appendix A) for more information on the disease and the test.

Porphyria

Porphyria is a metabolic disease whose symptoms include photosensitivity and the excretion of porphyrins in the urine. Porphyrins form the basis for hemoglobin, chlorophyll, and some enzymes. A high-carbohydrate, low-fat, low-protein diet helps a sufferer lead a normal life, as long as he also avoids barbiturates, penicillin, sulfa drugs, birth control pills, and chloroquine.

SOME OTHER CAUSES

Before accepting a final verdict of schizophrenia—or Alzheimer's—you should also look into the following possible contributing factors or causes. They, like everything before, are easily diagnosed and treated.

Depression

According to Dr. Reading, in *Your Family Tree Connection,* depression can be inherited. If you have red-green color blindness, you should especially look into this possibility: red-green color blindness is an X-linked genetic marker indicating a predisposition toward depression.

Depression can also be a side effect of mercury poisoning and hypoglycemia. Exercise and a proper diet are the therapies here. Reread this book, paying special attention to the sections on "Exercise" (see page 92) and "Blood-Sugar Problems" (see below). In addition, read *Sugar Blues,* a book by William Dufty.

Brain Abnormalities

Dr. E. L. Merrin, in the *Journal of Nervous and Mental Disorders,* reports that 23 percent of the patients in a study were diagnosed as being psychotic but in reality had some kind of abnormality in their brain. The abnormalities included tumors, slow-growing lesions, blood clots, and abnormally developed congenital tissue.

Based on the results of this study, I strongly suggest that you also have a CAT scan before giving up all hope for recovery. A CAT scan will reveal these types of problems.

Blood-Sugar Problems

Many mental symptoms, especially depression, are caused by blood-sugar problems. Some low-blood-sugar reactions are allergic reactions to foods that do not contain any form of sugar at all. According to Dr. Carl C. Pfeiffer, in *Mental and Elemental Nutrients: A Physician's Guide to Nutrition and Health Care,* hypoglycemia indicates a manganese deficiency caused by eating too much junk food containing sugar and white flour. Most brain-fogged subjects have faulty sugar metabolism.

Diabetes—high blood sugar—when untreated, can cause blindness, heart disease, obesity, impotence, and other dangerous physical and psychiatric problems. Always be aware of what your body is trying to tell you. Diabetes is characterized by excessive thirst and urination. In the absence of diabetes, excessive urine excretion is an indication of mercury toxicity. Other symptoms pointing toward the possibility of diabetes are a weary, heavy feeling; depression; incessant chattering; and an inability to stay focused on one subject (scattered thought processes).

Whatever else your physician recommends, follow a regular exercise program. Don't fool around with diabetes; follow your doctor's orders! I have a twenty-six-year-old friend who was blinded by diabetes—in one day.

A QUICK WORD ABOUT NEUROSIS

Before we leave this chapter, let me just mention neurosis.

Neurosis is caused by dysfunctional familial behavior. Children have the right to expect the same behavior from their parents as they get from the schoolteachers they respect. A good example of healthy familial behavior is found in the book *To Kill a Mockingbird*, by Harper Lee. Unfortunately, many children are raised in a dysfunctional family that is not emotionally equipped to nurture them. The dysfunctional behavior is then replicated generation after generation, until the cycle is finally interrupted by the intervention of a smart psychologist.

The best way to know if you need the services of a psychologist is if you recognize any destructive, self-defeating patterns in your actions or relationships. Instead of remaining in an unhealthy situation, you can learn to take responsibility for the only thing you can change or really control: yourself. In so doing, you create your own destiny.[3]

Every person in the world probably feels guilty about something in his past, or angry about the hand in life he was dealt. Often, the better a person is, the more guilty he feels. This is the norm. Few parents are sensitive, loving, and caring enough not to evoke any anger in their children. Many times, they send mixed signals to their offspring, who accept everything at face value. Most parents teach their children to "do as I say, not as I do," which distorts or twists the children's value systems.

You may well ask why I mention neurosis in a book about Alzheimer's disease. The answer is that chemicals seem to affect the same parts of the brain in neurosis as in mixed-up thought processes, blowing feelings out of proportion to reality. In addition, some people bury their feelings about traumatic experiences beyond their conscious thought, causing themselves unhappiness, depression, and all sorts of problems in life—including tremendous stress on their immune system.

For people from a dysfunctional family background, psychotherapy can, at times, be very painful. It's tough facing your problems. If you are having emotional problems, find a very smart psychologist. Make a friend you never knew you had: yourself. Become all that you can.[4]

Schizophrenia—physical sister, I believe, and soul sister to Alzheimer's—is a very scary affliction, for victim and family alike. Progress is being made, however. With the fields of allergy and nutrition making headway by leaps and bounds today, the mysterious causes and then obvious cures will all soon be uncovered. As with Alzheimer's, spirit is the key—a fighting spirit. Schizophrenia and Alzheimer's can be conquered. I did it. You can, too.

Conclusion

When I first realized how many actions I would have to take, how much information I would have to learn, and how many lifestyle changes I would have to make in order to recover, I was overwhelmed, as are all cerebral-allergy patients. There are so many habits to change and things to give up. Believe me, however, that in a year, you will feel so much better than you do now, you will wonder why you ever considered these changes to be a challenge. Just do one thing at a time, starting preferably with the clean room.

This book would be pointless if I didn't admonish you to stay the course and take charge of your treatment as much as possible. Either do the things that are good for your body and will therefore improve your health; or refuse to make the necessary changes to relieve your stress, improve your diet, and rebuild your body, and continue in the stagnation and decline of your health.

Unfortunately, there is no magic pill that will return you to health the easy way, which is what allopathic Alzheimer's researchers are spending hundreds of millions of dollars seeking. The hard fact is that no one but *you* can save you. Doctors can help you take the first few steps in the beginning, and your family can help a great deal during the middle stages of recovery. But in the later stages, when you start feeling fairly well and your mind begins to clear, you must take over completely. This is when it is most difficult to stay the course because you feel fine again and think you can bend a few rules once in a while. But you must not stray. You must stick to your diet and vitamin therapy, and stay away from allergens, or you will slip back into Alzheimer's, possibly beyond help. The lifestyle changes we're talking about here are *lifelong*. But they are also *life-giving*.

One of my doctors told me that people with a lot of brain allergies have a difficult time sticking with the rules. This seems to be true. A nurse once told me about a woman who continued to eat the foods to which she was allergic and who eventually slipped into irreversible Alzheimer's. Others who were perhaps just as ill—me included—have, within reason, recovered. Some of us now have challenging careers and a satisfying, happy life. I have even met a cerebral-allergy subject who returned to robust health in six months. Even though his job required him to eat many of his meals in restaurants, he maintained his good health.

A DOCTOR BY ANY OTHER NAME

One of the most important things you can do for yourself is to find physicians who are familiar with the treatment processes discussed in this book. Your local allergy or Dental Amalgam Syndrome (DAMS) group will be your best source of information. (See Appendices A and B.) Many of the authors I read while trying to figure out how to help myself referred to particular physicians in a manner indicating they were pre-eminent in their field. I contacted the physicians most often mentioned and became their patient.

Do not expect traditional (allopathic) physicians, even traditional allergists, to be familiar with, or to give adequate and unbiased advice about, clinical ecologists, orthomolecular psychiatrists, homeopathic physicians, naturopathic physicians, and dental detoxicologists and their treatments. No real communication seems to exist between the traditional medical community and alternative-practice physicians. The majority of alternative-practice physicians were originally allopathic practitioners before developing an interest in chronic disease, for which, they discovered, their traditional medical training offers few answers.

While searching for physicians to help you back to health, keep in mind that medical specialists are generally unfamiliar with areas of medical knowledge outside their immediate practice, the same way a life-insurance salesman is unfamiliar with group health insurance or a criminal attorney is unfamiliar with corporate law. They all carry a general title—physician, attorney, insurance salesman—but each tends to lack in-depth knowledge of the fields outside his specialty. Try to use a medical specialist only within his field of expertise.

Also keep in mind that the word "patient" is a highfalutin substitute for the word "customer." The words "patient" and "client" make doctors and other professionals sound more noble. But if you think of yourself as a customer, it puts you in control, with the doctor—or lawyer or other professional—a vendor who's just selling you his services. No matter how sophisticated and professional your doctor seems to be, you are the better judge of what's best for you and how well a treatment is working, not the other way around.

Many years ago, a friend on his death bed gave me

some advice about doctors that has been very helpful to me. In fact, it saved me a bundle in medical fees and probably saved my life. His advice? When you realize that healing is not progressing favorably, it's time to switch doctors and try another approach.

BACK TO THE BASICS

There will be times when you cannot maintain control of your health regimen no matter what you do; when you seem to be in complete compliance, yet the problems still arise. This is a particularly disappointing time.

When this happens—and it happens to everyone—go *back to the basics.* Retire to your clean room until your thinking clears and you feel good again. And think. Think about what new item may have been brought into your environment just before you seemed to fall apart. Has the pollen season started? Has some chemical recently been applied inside or outside your home?

Are you rotating your foods? What new foods are you eating? Check food labels for chemical additives or colorings. Do you cook with gas? Are you using a new cosmetic? Have you changed your vitamins?

An engineer I know built a beautiful, uncontaminated house that was delightful to visit—until he applied a sealer, advertised to be environmentally safe, to the ceiling. He has been suffering from asthma ever since. In fact, I have asthma for several days after visiting his home. The man's thoughtful disposition and health have now both deteriorated as a result of his allergy flare-up. Yet he remains unable to associate the sealer with his declining health.

Normally, my friend should have been able to protect himself by smelling the new sealer before applying it. Unfortunately, he also has a medical complication that prevents him from detecting odors. *The nose is the first line of defense for cerebral-allergy patients.*

After applying fifty-four gallons of a deck sealer, an acquaintance of another friend subsequently developed cancer and died. The subject's oncology physicians said they suspected the cancer was related to the sealer. If common household sealers are suspected of causing such a devastating disease as cancer, maybe it's time to suspect all chemical odors. Think about it. By the time your nose has detected an odor, the toxic chemical that is out-gassing is simultaneously being transferred into your bloodstream through your lungs. When people expose their bodies to chemical contamination, their tissues are no less susceptible to degeneration than the too-soft salmon caught near Seattle that the Anacortes cannery rejected, as I mentioned in Chapter 3. People's livers are just as susceptible to pollution as the little cougar's—and maybe more. Wild animals probably eat more wholesome food than people do. At the least, they don't eat junk food. And they certainly exercise more.

Remember the rules. They're to free you, not restrict you. If you are having trouble with your memory, have a friend remember. A woman bitterly complained to me that she was miserable even though she was carefully abiding by all the rules she had had to learn as a hospitalized clinical ecology patient. To reinforce her story, she displayed a jug of spring water she had purchased for drinking in order to avoid chlorine. The container was plastic. She had been through the same clinical ecology program that I had, but she forgot about using synthetic substances.

We all forget now and then. When you do, and you start feeling ill, go *back to the basics*. Nothing else works. Remember the three legs of the milking stool. Join a local allergy support group. Carefully study all the books I have listed. If necessary, read the books outside, in a breeze.

Save and reread this book many times. Your reading, along with your close contact with your allergy support group, will be your fastest, easiest way to learn what you must do to protect yourself. It will be your surest route to recovery.

Good luck on your journey!

Appendix A

For Referrals and Information

The following organizations can answer your questions, plus help you find knowledgeable physicians, dental detoxicologists, and allergy groups in your area.

American Academy of
  Environmental Medicine
P.O. Box 16106
Denver, CO 80216
(303) 622-9755

American Association of
  Orthomolecular Physicians
900 North Federal Highway
Suite 330
Boca Raton, FL 33432
(407) 393-6167

Canadian Schizophrenia
  Foundation
7375 Kingsway
Burnaby, BC V3N 3B5
Canada
(604) 521-1728

Canadian Society for
  Environmental Medicine
John G. Maclennan, M.D.
(416) 682-8241
(Please contact by phone
  only)

Foundation for Toxic Free
  Dentistry
P.O. Box 608010
Orlando, FL 32860-8010
(Please contact by mail
  only)

Princeton BioCenter
862 Route 518
Skillman, NJ 08588
(609) 924-8607

Toxic Element Research
  Foundation
P.O. Box 2589
Colorado Springs, CO 80901
(800) 331-2303

Well Mind Association
4649 Sunnyside Avenue
  North
Seattle, WA 98103
(206) 547-6167

Appendix B
DAMS
Coordinators

The following people are the coordinators for the state Dental Amalgam Syndrome (DAMS) groups. Write to them for information on your local chapter, or for referrals to knowledgeable physicians, dental detoxicologists, and allergy groups. Please contact the coordinators by mail only.

Alaska DAMS
Bob Stephenson
1837 No Way Lane
Fairbanks, AK 99079-6338

Arizona DAMS
Virginia Brown
405 North Granada
Tucson, AZ 85701

California DAMS
Dallas Pattee
38889 Road 108
Cutler, CA 93615

Colorado DAMS
Shirley Brown
P.O. Box 19032
Denver, CO 80219

Florida DAMS
Joanne Laskowski, R.N.
412-C Southwest 69th Street
Gainesville, FL 32607

Georgia DAMS
Glenda B. Smith
1270 Bridgewater Walk
Snellville, GA 30278

Illinois DAMS
Louise Herbeck
P.O. Box 9065
Downers Grove, IL 60515

Indiana DAMS
Pat House
10230 Saint Road 38-E
Lafayette, IN 47905

Michigan DAMS
Carolyn Smith
426 Grant
Grand Haven, MI 49417
or
Michigan DAMS
Marilyn Kiefer, R.N.
23272 North Rosedale Court
Saint Clair Shores, MI 48080

New Mexico DAMS
Murine Brake
725-9 Tramway Lane
  Northeast
Albuquerque, NM 87122

New York DAMS
Anita Karimian, Ph.D.
P.O. Box 1136
Madison Square Garden
New York, NY 10159

North Carolina DAMS
Pat Preyer
P.O. Box 11561
Winston-Salem, NC 27106
or
North Carolina DAMS
Bernice Rudelick
8313 Pineville-Matthews
  Road
Charlotte, NC 28226

Pennsylvania DAMS
Carol Ward
7426 Rhoads Street
Philadelphia, PA 19151

Tennessee DAMS
Mary F. Fox
5615 Orchard Road
Knoxville, TN 37919

Texas DAMS
Wanda Ballew
P.O. Box 342
Portland, TX 78374

Washington DAMS
Cheryl Quackenbush, R.N.
1617 First Street #19
Kirkland, WA 98033

Appendix C

For More Information

For more information on the topics discussed in this book, please contact the following.

Russ Borneman, D.D.S.
Burton Building
Suite 211
Anacortes, WA 98221
(206) 293-8451

Sandra Denton, M.D.
Huggins Diagnostic, Inc.
P.O. Box 2589
Colorado Springs, CO 80901
(800) 331-2303

International Health
  Foundation
P.O. Box 1000
Jackson, TN 38302

Hal A. Huggins, D.D.S., M.S.
Huggins Diagnostic, Inc.
P.O. Box 2589
Colorado Springs, CO 80901
(800) 331-2303

Northwest Healing Arts
  Center
13401 Bel-Red Road
Bellevue, WA 98005
(206) 747-9200

Overeaters Anonymous
P.O. Box 92870
Los Angeles, CA 90009
(213) 542-8363

United Farm Workers
 of America
P.O. Box 62, La Paz
Keene, CA 93531
(805) 822-5571

Appendix D

Product Information

To purchase the products mentioned in this book, please contact the following suppliers. Also listed are some items that are not discussed in the book but that are helpful to Alzheimer's sufferers.

CHAPTER 2

To order any of the books written by Dr. Patrick Störtebecker, please write to the Störtebecker Foundation for Research, Åkerbyuägen 282, S-183 35 Täby/Stockholm, Sweden.

Detoxosode, a homeopathic dental remedy to remove plastics and metals from the body, is available from Ho Bon, 3200 Polaris Avenue, Las Vegas, NV 89102. Do not drink coffee for at least two weeks before taking a homeopathic remedy. In addition, do not use an electric blanket, go to the dentist, or eat spicy foods. All four actions will act as an antidote.

Health Consciousness is an excellent magazine for anyone interested in better health. It is published by Roy Kupsinel, M.D., P.O. Box 550, Oviedo, FL 32765; (407) 365-6681.

CHAPTER 3

Environmental Purification Systems sells vacuum reading boxes. Contact the company at P.O. Box 191, Concord, CA 94552; (415) 284-2129.

Computer monitor filters to reduce radiation and glare from computer screens are available from Sun-Flex P.L., 1556 Halford Avenue, Santa Clara, CA 95051; (408) 522-8550. In Washington State and Oregon, contact Scott Figueroa at (206) 882-1392.

Nigra Enterprises can be reached at (818) 889-6877. The owner, Jim Nigra, is an extremely knowledgeable, helpful filter salesman. He also sells hexametaphosphate, which whitens white clothes beautifully in place of chlorine.

Clean Sip, according to Global Star Products, is "the world's smallest water filter in a straw." It is described as long-lasting, portable, and reusable, and filters out chlorine, lead, mercury, hydrogen, aluminum, arsenic, cadmium, chromium, algae, fungus, scale, and sediment. In Canada, contact Global Star Products at 67 Steelcase Road West, Unit 4, Toronto (Markham), ON L3R 2M4; (416) 470-7460. In the United States, the company can be reached at Suite 109, 10101 South Western, Oklahoma City, OK 73139; (405) 634-6096.

Mine Safety Appliances sells Dustfoe 66 and Dustfoe 77 masks. To order, call (800) MSA-2222. Keep the mask in an airtight plastic bag when not in use to prevent dust and pollens from contaminating it. When it does get dirty, it can be disassembled for thorough washing. Hint: order fifty extra filters.

To purchase Amway products, check your phone book for your local distributors.

Community Mattress, Concord, CA 94520, sells cotton mattresses. The phone number is (415) 798-9785.

RCI Environmental sells formaldehyde testing kits. Contact the company at 2701 West 15th Street, Suite 250, Plano, TX 75075; (214) 596-8749.

Debra Lynn Dadd has written an excellent book, *Nontoxic and Natural: How to Avoid Dangerous Everyday Products and Buy or Make Safe Ones,* that discusses which products are safe for allergy sufferers. The book costs $14.95 and can be ordered from P.O. Box 279, Forest Knowls, CA 94933; (800) 488-3233. (The phone number is for Visa and MasterCard orders only.)

Super Blue-Green Algae can be obtained from Super Blue-Green Algae, 1006 Wagon Wheel Gap Road, Boulder, CO 80302; (800) 347-5506 (United States and Canada).

Perque vitamin and mineral supplements can be obtained from Perk People, 862 Route 518, Rocky Hill, NJ 08558; (800) 553-5472.

The Crystal Deodorant Stone, says its manufacturer, is "300 percent more effective than commercial deodorants but 100 percent pure and natural." It lasts for months, contains no aluminum, and only needs to be used once every seven to ten days. You can purchase it from Leon, Box 224, 253 College Street, Toronto, ON M5T 1R5, Canada; (416) 462-6557.

CHAPTER 4

Phenols are being called "a new treatment process with great promise." At present, there are probably less

than fifty physicians who are familiar with the new phenolic process for desensitizing food allergies that cross food
family lines. With the process, you don't need more than
fourteen different desensitizing medications, for no more
than seven weeks, to abolish bad reactions to foods. This is
especially welcome news to people with multiple food
allergies. The Well Mind Association, 4649 Sunnyside
Avenue North, Seattle, WA 98103, has three papers available on phenolic food compounds. The cost is $1.50 per
copy.

- *Use of Phenylated Food Compounds in Diagnosis and
  Treatment of 100 Patients With Food Allergy and Phe-
  nol Intolerance,* by J. J. McGovern, Jr., M.D.; R. W.
  Gardiner, Ph.D.; and L. D. Brenneman, M.D., Ph.D.
- *Basic Chemistry of Allergens,* by Robert W. Gardiner,
  Ph.D., professor of Animal Science, Brigham Young
  University, Provo, Utah.
- *CNS Effect of Phenyl Compounds in Food,* by J. J.
  McGovern, Jr., M.D., and R. W. Gardiner, Ph.D.

Appendix E

The
PAR Booklet

Proper Amalgam Removal

Avoiding the
"Frying Pan Into the Fire"
Syndrome

Prepared by

Huggins Diagnostic, Inc.

Contents

ICBM Declaration

The International Conference on the Biocompatibility of Materials

declares that:

"Based on the known toxic potentials of mercury and its documented release from dental amalgams, usage of mercury-containing amalgam increases the health risk of the patients, the dentists, and dental personnel."

The above statement is a landmark conclusion for dentistry. It demonstrates the key concept which is the focus of this booklet: The individual biocompatibility of a material should be fully evaluated before it is placed within a patient.

The ICBM Declaration was not entered into lightly. It is the result of the total ICBM Conference which was jointly sponsored by the University of Colorado at Colorado Springs and the Toxic Element Research Foundation during the week of November 5–10, 1988. Dr. Douglas Swartzendruber, an experimental pathologist with Colorado University, and Dr. Hal A. Huggins, General Director of the Toxic Element Research Foundation, were co-chairmen of the Conference.

Twenty-four major speakers representing research efforts from around the world made presentations at the ICBM Conference. Research was presented pertinent to the health risks surrounding the use of restorative materials in medicine and dentistry. Specific topics included toxicology, biocompatibility of materials currently in use, effects by these materials in the

brain and nervous system, psychological reactions me-
diated by materials exposure, immunologic, muta-
genic, and teratologic data, as well as risk assessment
considerations.

Included among the presenters were the following:

Duane Cutright, DDS, Ph.D., Keynote Speaker
–Former Chief of Oral Pathology for the US Army
Institute of Dental Research at the Walter Reed
Army Hospital

Louis Chang, Ph.D.
–Director of Interdisciplinary Toxicology and Experi-
mental Pathology, and Professor of Pathology &
Toxicology at the University of Arkansas

Klas Nordlind, MD, Ph.D.
–Assistant Professor for the Department of Der-
matology at the Karolinska Hospital in Stockholm,
Sweden

Magnus Nylander, DDS, Ph.D. Cand.
–Research scientist with the Karolinska Institute in
Stockholm, Sweden

Vladmir Bencko, MD, Ph.D., D.Sc.
–Postgraduate School of Medicine in Prague, Czechoslovakia

Max Costa, Ph.D.
–Vice Chairman of the Department of Environmental
Medicine at the New York University Medical Cen-
ter and Professor of Pharmacology at NYU Medical
Center

Patrick Exbrayat, DDS, MS, Ph.D. Cand.
–Faculte d'Odontologie de Lyon Department of
Dental Materials and Assistant Professor at Lyon
University in Lyon, France

Frederick Berglund, MD, Ph.D.
 –Research scientist investigating the dangers of materials used in dentistry; Stockholm, Sweden

Mats Hanson, Ph.D.
 –Research scientist investigating the dangers of materials used in dentistry; Veberod, Sweden

Horst Poehlmann, MBBS, Ph.D.
 –Private medical practice and research in Adelaide, Australia

Joel R. Butler, Ph.D.
 –Professor of Psychology at the University of North Texas

Sandra Denton, MD
 –Private medical practice with the Johnathan Wright Clinic in Seattle, WA

Mike Godfrey, MBBS
 –Private medical practice and research in Mt. Maunganui, New Zealand

Jean Monro, MD
 –Private medical practice and research in London, England

Graeme Ewers, BDSc, Ph.D.
 –Adjunct Professor at the University of Western Australia in Perth, Australia

Zane Gard, MD
 –Private medical practice in San Diego, California

Paul Slovic, Ph.D.
 –President of Decision Research and Former President of the Society for Risk Analysis at the University of Oregon in Eugene, Oregon

Robert Sibelrud, OD, MS, Ph.D. Cand.
  –Ph.D. Candidate at Colorado State University and private practice in Fort Collin, CO

Sam Wong, Jr., DDS
  –University of Hawaii and private dental practice in Honolulu, Hawaii

Anthony Newbury, MDS, LDS
  –Private dental practice in London, England

Douglas Swartzendruber, Ph.D.
  –Associate Professor for the Department of Biology at Colorado University at Colorado Springs

Hal A. Huggins, DDS, MS
  –MS at the University of Colorado at Colorado Springs and General Director of the Toxic Element Research Foundation

Video presentations in absentia and presentation with permission by delegation at the Conference:

Leonard T. Kurlund, MD, Ph.D.
  –Department of Health Sciences Research Section of Clinical Epidemiology for the Mayo Clinic in Rochester, MN

Olympio Pinto, DDS, MS
  –Private dental practice and research in Rio de Janeiro

Banquet Speaker

In addition Colonel James Irwin, Apollo 15 Astronaut and Moon walker, was the featured Banquet speaker.

Introduction

Dentists have debated the safety of amalgam as a restorative since the 1830s when amalgam was first introduced in the United States. A more detailed discussion of the amalgam problem is presented in Chapter One of this booklet. At this time, however, it should be noted that many dentists are in a quandary when they encounter patients who want their amalgams replaced.

Considering the state of the profession, the confusion of the average dentist is understandable.

First, dental leadership argues that it is "unhealthy" for dentists to remove amalgam for health reasons. In other words, if the dentist removes amalgams out of concern that the mercury in amalgam may jeopardize the patient's health, dental leadership considers this "unethical." Not only is this a general problem for dentists across the nation, but in several states dental leadership has taken the unusual position of threatening to censure dentists who inform their patients that amalgam contains mercury.

However, if the patient and doctor agree that the amalgam fillings are unattractive, dental leadership then argues that a dentist may ethically replace the amalgams.

We view the present position of dental leadership with grave concern. It is our view that national legislation banning amalgam is required. Sadly, such legislation is unlikely until the public—the fathers, mothers, men, and women of the United States—raise an outcry of intense concern to their state and national legislators.

We hope that the readers of this booklet will participate in such a movement.

There is a positive note to this unhealthy situation, however. Replacement dental materials for amalgam do exist which more closely resemble the natural appearance of the tooth. This is certainly to be desired since amalgams over time turn black, and—even when they are first placed—do not look anything like the natural tooth.

We are much more concerned with the patient's health. But it would appear, at least, that dentists and patients who desire amalgam removal should simply observe that "amalgams are ugly."

But a second and much more serious reason for confusion about proper amalgam removal (PAR) exists. Simply put, it is that most dentists are unfamiliar with the protocol recommended by Dr. Huggins. Consequently, the average dentist is unlikely to provide body chemistry testing, nutritional and dietary counseling, specific supplementation, sequential removal of fillings, or proper serum compatibility testing.

And as a result, the patient who has amalgams replaced without consideration for these procedures is in danger of ending up worse—sometimes, much worse—rather than better.

This is what we refer to as the "frying pan into the fire" syndrome.

And the tragedy is that some patients—either through ignorance or in an effort to save money by omitting required steps—literally go from the "frying pan into the fire." But trying to ignore the possible consequences of the "syndrome" is like playing Russian roulette. The results can be devastating, and in some cases, irreversible.

In line with this, we get numerous phone calls each day from patients who have either accidentally or intentionally omitted the steps in proper amalgam removal (PAR). These patients report a variety of resulting complications. Some have gone into shock, some have thrown premature ventricular contractions (PVC's), some have been hospitalized, and some have been placed in mental institutions.

Understandably, we are extremely concerned that patients go through *all* of the proper protocol. The patient needs health care that's up to par, and from our perspective "par" is "proper amalgam removal."

Those who desire a more thorough treatment of the amalgam problem will find it in *It's All in Your Head,* the *Annotated Bibliography,* and Dr. Huggins' thesis on the toxicity of amalgam components and the regulatory agencies which govern these components. *The PAR Booklet* itself is an overview and a step-by-step guide detailing the required procedures.

As a result, the prospective patient is strongly encouraged to carefully read this booklet, and to act upon the information that is presented within the booklet's pages.

One

What Is the Problem?

Amalgam Fillings: Cause for Concern

You wouldn't give your child a leaky thermometer, because mercury is a poison; nor would you put a poison in your child's mouth. . . .

But your dentist does.

These are alarming words, but they present a real problem which faces your family and which also faces you as an individual.

Mercury is one of the oldest recognized and strongest poisons known to man. And yet the amalgam—the commonly used silver filling—is an average of 52% pure mercury.

A Brief Amalgam History

Historically, Alice, of Wonderland fame, brought the Mad Hatter to our attention. Although the work was obviously fiction, this character was based on fact. Hatters who used mercury compounds in the shaping of felt hats were observed to have strange mental quirks which were termed "madness."

But dentists have placed amalgam fillings for over 150 years; why would they do this if the material is poisonous?

The answer to this lies in economics and history.

When amalgam was originally introduced in the United States around 1830, the then National Dental

Association sternly warned against its use. The alternative material at that time, however, was gold; and amalgam as a cheaper, easier to use restorative gained popular acceptance in the dental profession.

Mercury Leaches Out of Amalgams

Over the course of the years the dental profession has argued that mercury remains bound within amalgam fillings and does not come out. And yet studies—especially over the last twenty years—indicate that as much as 180 micrograms of mercury per day leach out of the fillings and potentially into the patient's body. More to the point, one researcher reported a direct relationship between the number of amalgam fillings in cadavers and the amount of mercury accumulated in their brains.

How important is this quantity of mercury to you?

A preliminary study performed at Colorado University in Colorado Springs showed that mercury in the ratio of less than 40 parts per billion was lethal to white blood cells. Another Colorado University study reported that live bone cells were killed by mercury in concentrations as small as 0.4 parts per million. And yet it is estimated that there is at least 700 times more mercury than this resting in gum tissue next to mercury-silver (amalgam) fillings.

In addition, researchers have reported changes in bodily function such as conditioned reflexes, thyroid uptake, heart ECG, liver function, adrenal gland activity, and immunologic responses at mercury exposure levels of only 10 to 30 micrograms per day. Even more dramatic is the study which reports changes in conditioned reflexes at mercury concentrations as low as 2 to 5 micrograms per day.

Consider these statistics in light of the fact that the Toxic Element Research Foundation estimates that the amount of daily mercury exposure from just one average amalgam is in excess of 3 micrograms per day.

But an even more frightening aspect of mercury poisoning from amalgam is its effect on the unborn.

Mercury swiftly passes through the placental barrier and accumulates in the fetal blood at levels up to 30% higher than in the mother. More to the point, in these situations mercury appears to be especially injurious to the central nervous system of infants and children. And beyond this, of the total mercury in the fetus, 19 times more mercury accumulates in the fetal brain than proportionately accumulates in the mother's brain.

What Mercury Can Do in Your Body

But what conditions follow mercury exposure from amalgam?

Habitual exposure to even very small amounts of mercury has been associated with a variety of symptoms. In a survey of 1,320 patients evaluated by the Huggins Diagnostic Center, the following frequency of symptoms was reported:

• 73% reported chronic irritability.
• 72% indicated they suffered chronic depression.
• 67% manifested numbness and tingling of the extremities.
• 63% reported unexplained chronic fatigue.
• 58% indicated difficulty in memory functions.
• 55% manifested sudden, unexplained anger.
• 54% reported difficulty in making routine decisions.
• 37% admitted to suicidal thoughts.

But this is just the beginning of the problem.

Virtually everyone reacts to the presence of mercury. This universal reaction, however, is not easily seen in all people who have mercury-silver fillings. Only some people react strongly enough to require medical help. Unfortunately, this medical help is usually unsuccessful as long as mercury remains in the body.

And what diseases are associated with those who react?

Briefly there are five divisions of disease reported to improve with amalgam removal. They are:

1. Neurological—including emotional responses such as depression, anxiety, and irritability as well as neural effects such as facial twitches, muscle spasms, epilepsy and multiple sclerosis.
2. Cardiovascular effects—unexplained rapid heart rate and/or unidentified chest pains.
3. Collagen diseases—such as lupus, arthritis, and scleroderma.
4. Immunologic effects—lowering the body's defense system capacity and the viability of white blood cells.
5. Allergies—mercury can alter chemistries so that some people become sensitive to foods and chemicals.

The Threshold Concept

Again, not all patients come down with identifiable diseases as a result of mercury contamination from amalgams. However, mercury will diminish immune system effectiveness. And this in turn is related to what Dr. Huggins calls the "threshold concept."

Generally, the body's immune system has multiple avenues of defense against any given body chemistry offense. As a result, numerous negative factors may be introduced into a patient's system without the development of obvious disease. Somewhere in life's experiences—depending on the patient's stamina and immune mechanisms—the "straw that breaks the camel's back" may be introduced. At that point a seemingly minor immune challenge may result in the onset of a serious medical condition.

It is at this point that threshold is reached and the last defense mechanism gives out. This is like walking towards a cliff with a two thousand foot drop. While you're walking toward the cliff, everything seems fine. Your steps are the same as always and nothing appears to be out of the ordinary. But when you take that last step and fall down the two thousand foot drop, things change for the worse in a hurry.

Again, heavy metal contamination from dental materials can play a part in this threshold phenomenon. The ongoing accumulation of mercury from amalgam can move the patient toward threshold. Subsequent exposure to additional heavy metal contaminants from dentistry and other sources can additionally weaken the body's defense systems.

When threshold is reached (and the patient "steps over the cliff") serious problems can arise. The frightening thing about the process is that it is difficult to analyze just how close any given patient is to "the cliff."

Since contamination from dental materials is suspect in this problem, prudence dictates caution in the dental process. And yet the current dental leadership does not even acknowledge that the problem exists.

The Bottom Line

How serious is this problem?

Recent research by the Toxic Element Research Foundation demonstrated that at least 90% of the subjects tested had already developed immune responses to mercury. This result is certainly not surprising in a population exposed to mercury from amalgam.

But not all of the test subjects had symptoms which warranted medical treatment. Over time, however, needless ongoing exposure to mercury is capable of taking its toll.

And who will be affected?

Men? Women? Children? The unborn child?

Perhaps you will be affected.

The important thing, however, is not how many will be affected.

The bottom line is that mercury should not be placed in the mouth at all if even just a few percent (let alone 90%) of the population already shows a reaction to it.

Two

What Is the Solution?

What Not to Do

Do *not* have your amalgams removed without going through *all* the steps!

Dr. Huggins' book, entitled *It's All in Your Head*, gives the above emphatic warning on page 110. It is a warning which is all too frequently ignored by patients to their own detriment.

There are acceptable alternatives to amalgam, but these alternatives need to be determined on a patient by patient basis (through proper serum compatibility testing). There is no one material which is safe for all people. Consequently, amalgam replacement needs to be approached with all the proper steps in their proper sequence.

Again, we want to emphasize that Huggins Diagnostic Center receives numerous calls each day from patients who have violated this warning, had their amalgams removed without following the complete protocol, and who are now worse than before. In line with this, we have had patients report that they have gone into shock, that they have thrown premature ventricular contractions (PVC's), or that they have ended up in the hospital or mental institution—all because they haven't gone through the necessary steps.

It is essential to bear in mind that improperly performed or omitted procedures may permanently alter chemistries. Consequently, recovery from amalgam toxicity is like trying to make a strike in bowling. The bowler only gets one chance to make his strike, and the patient may only have one opportunity to properly deal with his health problem.

Remember, the actual dentistry is the last of a series of steps in the required protocol. The dentistry itself is like firing a loaded gun. The preliminary steps of loading and carefully aiming the gun must be taken before the trigger is pulled (that is, before the dentistry is performed). Obviously, once the "bullet" has been fired, you can't get it back.

Three Initial Steps

The steps themselves are relatively simple to follow.

1. Contact a Patient Advisor at Huggins Diagnostic Center (800-331-2303 or 719-473-4703).
2. Your Patient Advisor will encourage you to read the book *It's All in Your Head.*
3. Your Patient Advisor will present the two programs available through our office which are designed to help the mercury toxic patient. These programs are the Complete Assist Program and the In-Office Program.

   • The In-Office Program is for the patient whose health problems are serious.
   • The Complete Assist Program is for the patient whose health is adequate to work with our office "at a distance."

Required Laboratory Testing

Monitoring and adjusting patient chemistries through laboratory testing, dietary considerations, and specific

supplementation are critical parts of the required protocol. Consequently, whether you choose to become
an In-Office patient, or whether you work with us "at a
distance" through the Complete Assist Program, the
same foundational laboratory tests are required.
Therefore, the steps to take after you have accomplished the three listed above are:

4. Arrange for the required tests and procedures
    through your Patient Advisor (800-331-2303 or
    719-473-4703):

    • A "hair" analysis (trace mineral analysis).
    • A urine mercury analysis (atomic absorption
      testing with analysis of both organic and in-
      organic mercury).
    • A CBC/blood profile.
    • Completion of a *Mercury Toxicity Diagnosis and
      Nutritional Evaluation Questionnaire.*

The laboratory tests and questionnaire are the basis
for the Assist Report, a personalized 50-plus page report provided to both Complete Assist Program and In-
Office patients. The report presents your recommended nutritional and supplementation program.
For the In-Office patient these recommendations are
augmented and further adapted through personal consultation with Dr. Huggins.

A modified diet and specific supplementation in
accordance with Dr. Huggins' recommendations are
two of the major components in the required protocol.
Failure to implement proper diet and supplementation
guidelines per the Assist Report are significant road-
blocks to success in dealing with amalgam toxicity. In
line with this, it should be kept in mind that supple-

mentation is most effective when initiated two weeks prior to amalgam removal.

5. Arrange for Proper Serum Compatibility testing through your Patient Advisor (800-331-2303 or 719-473-4703). Proper Serum Compatibility testing helps determine which materials will be acceptable amalgam replacements in consideration of your specific health needs.

Adequate Dental Treatment

6. Arrange for a dental referral through your Patient Advisor (800-331-2303 or 719-473-4703). Dentists who practice the required protocol will incorporate the following into their treatment plan:

    *   The book *It's All in Your Head* as a basis for patient education.
    *   The required laboratory tests as a basis for the Assist Report.
    *   The Assist Report as a basis for individualized nutritional counseling and as a basis for specific supplementation.
    *   Proper Serum Compatibility testing from Huggins Diagnostic or CompatLabs.
    *   The sequential removal of fillings based upon electrical testing with an appropriate meter.
    *   The scheduling of dental appointments with appropriate consideration for patient immune cycles.
    *   The use of an air filtration system and/or an ion filtration (electrophoresis) system specifically designed to trap heavy metal contaminants such as mercury.

- The use of a rubber dam (where possible) during the dental procedures.

Follow Through With Follow-Up Testing

7. Arrange for follow-up testing and supplementation modification through your Patient Advisor (800-331-2303 or 719-473-4703). Follow-up testing should include:

   - A preliminary recall blood and urine test within three weeks to three months following amalgam removal.
   - A second recall to include a blood, hair and urine test six months after the preliminary recall.
   - Subsequent recall testing to be run at six month intervals as required by your health needs.

Summarizing the Steps

A summary of the seven steps listed above follows:

1. Contact a Patient Advisor (800-331-2303 or 719-473-4703).
2. Read *It's All in Your Head.*
3. Choose either the Complete Assist or the In-Office Program.
4. Make arrangements for the required tests and procedures.
5. Provide for Proper Serum Compatibility testing.
6. Prepare for adequate dental care.
7. Follow through with follow-up testing.

Three

The Initial Steps

Why All the Steps Are Important

A child pulling out the bottom container of a stack of soup cans at the grocery store quickly learns that there is an order in which some things must be done. So it is with amalgam toxicity therapy.

And more to the point, just as a bowler only gets one chance to make a strike, you may only get one chance to adequately deal with your health problems. Some steps—if done out of sequence or if performed improperly—may permanently alter your chemistries.

Let's consider the seven steps which are the required method.

Step One
Contacting a Patient Advisor

Contacting a Patient Advisor is the foundation for your treatment. Your Patient Advisor will aid you in coordinating your treatment program so that it is in accordance with the protocol developed by Dr. Huggins. A Patient Advisor can be reached by calling 800-331-2303 or 719-473-4703.

This is the logical place to start. And obviously, when dealing with the critical issue of personal health care, working with the expert is the key to getting the best help. Along this line, it is important to know that

Dr. Huggins is the pioneering researcher for amalgam toxicity therapy in America.

During the course of his work Dr. Huggins founded the Toxic Element Research Foundation. In addition, Dr. Huggins has fostered public awareness of the inherent dangers of amalgam toxicity through numerous television, radio, newspaper, and magazine interviews. Included in these interviews are sessions with nationally known media representatives such as Dan Rather, Gary Null, Tom Beardon, and David Horowitz. The *Sixty Minutes* affiliate in Australia produced a program on Dr. Huggins' work.

Interest in Dr. Huggins' work has led him to lecture in England, Germany, France, Czechoslovakia, Sweden and Denmark. In addition, Dr. Huggins has held seminars in New Zealand and Australia, and future plans include the Orient. Literally, Dr. Huggins is an internationally recognized authority on the subject of amalgam toxicity.

Further, Dr. Huggins has also completed a Master's Degree in Science with an emphasis in immunology at Colorado University in Colorado Springs. His Master's Thesis on the toxic and legal implications of amalgam components has created additional interest in the field.

But beyond this, his work and procedures are based on over twenty years of personal humanitarian effort with thousands of patients and doctors in the specific field of amalgam toxicity and heavy metal contamination from dental materials.

The goal of the Huggins Diagnostic Center Patient Advisor is to guide you through each step in the protocol developed by Dr. Huggins. Accordingly, the Patient Advisors are specifically trained to direct patients through the necessary procedures in this uniquely developed regimen. Consequently, the foundational step in the program is contacting a Patient Advisor (800-331-2303 or 719-473-4703).

Step Two
Reading *It's All in Your Head*

A well-informed patient is in a better position to obtain the treatment which will best meet his or her health needs. *It's All in Your Head* is the authoritative written compilation of the essential facts pertaining to the required protocol. Again, patients are better prepared to face the problems and potential solutions related to amalgam toxicity when they have a grasp of the necessary facts.

In addition, the book serves as a basis for informed interaction with the dentist. This can be a critical factor since most dentists (and even some who claim that they are personally trained by Dr. Huggins) deviate from the required protocol.

A word of caution is in order, however. The patient's needs are best served by reading the *entire* book and by diligently noting the instruction to go through *all* the required steps *before* amalgam removal.

The most frequent problem reported to the Huggins Diagnostic Center is that of the patient who—upon hearing of the potential dangers of mercury from amalgam—rushes out to have his amalgams replaced without the required protocol. Failure to go through the recommended steps of proper body chemistry analysis, nutritional evaluation, specific supplementation, compatibility testing (to determine acceptable replacement materials) or electrical testing (to determine sequential removal) can lead to needless complications.

People who have their amalgams removed without going through the required protocol can end up "jumping from the frying pan and into the fire."

Invariably these patients report that they are worse than ever. Such problems could be minimized by reading *It's All in Your Head* and then, with the help of a Patient Advisor, carefully applying the book's recommendations.

Step Three
Choosing the In-Office or the Complete Assist Program

There are only two health programs currently available which are based upon Dr. Huggins' protocol. Both are available by contacting a Patient Advisor at Huggins Diagnostic Center (800-331-2303 or 303-719-4703).

The Complete Assist Program is for the patient whose health problems are not serious and who can work with our office "at a distance." The In-Office Program is for the patient whose health problems are serious and who is able to travel to Colorado Springs for personal consultation with Dr. Huggins.

Both the Complete Assist and the In-Office Program are based upon basic laboratory tests (although Dr. Huggins frequently has more in-depth testing performed at Huggins Diagnostic Center for the In-Office patient). In addition, patients under both programs receive the Assist Report—a fifty-plus page compilation of standard counsel and personalized evaluation.

The In-Office patient, however, spends two to three days in consultation with Dr. Huggins and his staff. During the intensive counseling sessions, the Assist

Report recommendations and guidelines are further modified and augmented to meet the specific health requirements presented by the In-Office patient's chemistries and responses during the counseling sessions. In addition, the supplementation guidelines are "fine tuned" and the patient's program is monitored with an eye to even greater compliance with the required protocol.

The In-Office program also includes without further charge a preliminary telephone follow-up review. The patient, however, is responsible for the costs of the required lab work for this review. The review itself is routinely scheduled between three weeks and three months after amalgam removal.

Beyond this, the actual dentistry can be coordinated for the In-Office patient through the "bubble operatory"—a state-of-the-art dental facility specifically designed by Dr. Huggins to benefit the mercury toxic patient. Further, for the In-Office patient's convenience, Huggins Diagnostic Center can recommend nearby lodging which is available at a reasonable rate.

Both In-Office and Complete Assist patients receive without charge their first month's supply of recommended supplements. In-Office patients, however, receive additional prescription supplements—again without additional charge—which are not available to patients who elect to work with Dr. Huggins "at a distance."

The major factor for In-Office patient treatment, however, is personal attention. Typically, an In-Office patient spends time with a variety of support staff whose efforts are coordinated by Dr. Huggins. The support staff includes a nutritional counselor, a Feldenkrais practitioner, dental staff, laboratory staff, a general counselor and a Patient Advisor.

In addition, both In-Office and Complete Assist patients undergo compatibility testing as routine parts of their programs. And upon request the In-Office patient receives the further benefit of a Huggins Diagnostic staff member's personal review of the compatibility test recommendations with your dentist.

Again, the critical issues in deciding which program is best for you are the following two factors:

1.   The condition of your health.
2.   Your ability to travel to Huggins Diagnostic Center.

If your health problems are *serious* and you are able to travel to Huggins Diagnostic Center, then the In-Office Program is recommended for you.

If, on the other hand, your health problems are *not* serious and you are able to work with us "at a distance," then the Complete Assist Program will meet your needs.

The Bubble-Operatory

An additional benefit to the In-Office patient is the availability of the "bubble-op," a state-of-the-art dental operatory, designed by Dr. Huggins. The bubble-op incorporates a unique configuration that minimizes the accumulation of heavy metal contaminates. Included as part of the bubble-op hygienic control system are dual-activated charcoal air filters which continually sweep the operatory environment. An electrophoretic system attaches electrical charges to submicron and larger sized particles and then accumulates these charged particles at a collection plate. These combined processes purify the air.

In addition, the bubble-operatory is designed to

eliminate the out-gassing of formaldehyde. Specially constructed cabinets, sealed laminated surfaces and uniquely formulated paints and glues are used throughout the operatory with an eye to minimizing patient exposure.

The bubble-op also features a specially contoured dental chair, which adapts to the size of each patient. Perhaps the most outstanding aspect of the bubble-op is the opportunity for the patient to receive dentistry from a dentist who has direct on-going access to Dr. Huggins.

A further feature of the bubble-op is its innovative application of the Farady cage. The operatory's walls and ceilings contain a wire cage which totally surrounds the bubble operatory and is uniformly grounded. This structure has the effect of minimizing radiation and wavelengths at frequencies which may be harmful to the patient.

Patients interested in the bubble-op may arrange for scheduling by contacting their patient advisor at 800-331-2303 or 719-473-4703. Patients who use the bubble-op report that the combined hourly fee for dentistry and facility use is frequently comparable to specialty dentistry fees in their area.

The bubble-op is often used in cooperation with the patient's local dentist. Temporary materials may be the best option for some patients in order to stabilize their health until they return home. Following the stabilization period the patient's local dentist may be able to place more permanent materials.

Four

Testing and Procedures

Step Four
Making Arrangements for the Required
Tests and Procedures

Both the In-Office and the Complete Assist Programs require the same initial tests and procedures which your Patient Advisor will help you to obtain. In line with this, the following four items are required:

1. A "hair" analysis (trace mineral analysis).
2. A urine mercury analysis (atomic absorption testing, which analyzes both organic and inorganic mercury).
3. A CBC/blood profile.
4. Completion of a *Mercury Toxicity Diagnosis and Nutritional Evaluation Questionnaire.*

These items are the necessary elements in the construction of your Assist Report—a fifty-plus page compilation of standard counsel and personalized evaluation. To help understand this, consider your body's chemistry as if it were a shopper buying groceries at a supermarket. The bloodstream—which indicates materials available to the individual cells—would be represented by the supermarket. The hair—which indicates materials actually taken into the individual cells of your body—would be represented by the shopper's home pantry. Body chemistry analysis seeks to identify the materials "in the supermarket" as well as the materials "in the pantry."

In a simplified overview of these tests, then, the hair analysis is utilized as an indicator of specific materials taken into your body's cells. The urine mercury analysis, on the other hand, serves as a potential indicator of your body's mercury retention level.

The CBC is a separate test from the blood profile and is reported by many laboratories along with the blood profile report. The CBC is reviewed in your Assist Report as a potential indicator of immunologic function.

The blood profile, however, is evaluated for evidence about key materials which are available through the bloodstream for cell function. Whether or not these key materials in the bloodstream are actually incorporated in the cell chemistry is a matter of importance for body chemistry analysis. On the other hand, the *Mercury Toxicity Diagnosis and Nutritional Evaluation Questionnaire* serves as a "personal lifestyle" review and monitors a host of factors which could influence your health.

Again, these four items taken together are the required tests and procedures for your personalized Assist Report. Following below are key considerations in the actual test gathering procedures.

The Hair Analysis Specimen

The hair analysis should be performed on hair which is clean, which is *not* permed, and which is *not* dyed. Primarily for convenience purposes, the hair is best taken from the nape of the neck and should be cut as close to the scalp as possible. The use of thinning shears is recommended to keep the patient from looking "scalped."

For patients with longer hair, that portion which is more than two inches from the scalp should be cut and discarded. This is necessary in order to insure that the test result indicates "current" body chemistry activity rather than the activity of the body during prior periods.

Two tablespoons (one gram) of hair is necessary in order to process the hair specimen. Patients sending insufficient amounts of hair to the laboratory for testing can delay their test results by as much as five weeks.

Patients who lack head hair can use hair from other parts of the body. This is an acceptable, though not preferable, alternative since the laboratory test results are normed on head hair specimens.

The Urine Mercury Analysis Specimen

The specimen should be mailed to the laboratory in the padded, "bubble" mailer. The padded, "bubble" mailer may be obtained from Huggins Diagnostic Center along with a specially prepared 30-ml. urine tube. Mercury's tendency to bind to glass is impeded by silicon. Consequently, the urine tubes provided by Huggins Diagnostic Center are treated with a coating of silicon which is baked on.

In addition, the atomic absorption procedure requires a minimum 20-ml. specimen. Consequently the 30-ml. specimen container should be used.

Although the patient does not need to modify his or her diet for the urine mercury specimen, the specimen itself should *not* be taken from the first excretion of the day. Accordingly, specimens gathered from 10:00 A.M. to noon excretions are preferable.

The CBC/Blood Profile Specimen

The CBC/blood profile is actually two tests which are normally processed by laboratories on the same specimen. The specimen will be drawn by your doctor or local laboratory on "fasting" blood. A "fasting" blood specimen is most conveniently arranged by having the patient not eat any food nor drink anything but water from 8:00 P.M. of the evening *before* the day of the blood drawing. The specimen can then be drawn first thing the next morning.

It is important for the patient to drink a glass of water about fifteen minutes before the blood is drawn. This will insure that the tests are not run on "dehydrated" blood.

In addition, the CBC/blood profile should be ordered with a "Request for Laboratory Services" form which your Patient Advisor will help you to obtain. The request form instructs the laboratory to furnish the following results:

Serum Chemistry Profile
(must include the following)

calcium	phosphorous	glucose
cholesterol	triglycerides	uric acid
BUN	total protein	albumin
globulin	total bilirubin	alk phos
SGOT	LDH	

CBC With a Manual Differential
(must include the following)

red blood cell count	hemoglobin
eosinophils	basophils

reactive lymphs   neutrophils
actual platelet count   bands

Your local laboratory will give the requested CBC/ blood profile results to you, and you will send them to Huggins Diagnostic Center (P.O. Box 2589, Colorado Springs, CO 80901). These results become a part of your Assist Report and are compared with Dr. Huggins' "BCI" (Body Chemistry Ideal) values. In addition, these values are retained within the Huggins Diagnostic Center database for future comparison with your follow-up testing.

The BCI values represent ideal norms developed by Dr. Huggins through his research over several decades with thousands of patients. The BCI values are a narrower range than those conventionally used to evaluate an American population which is exposed to heavy metal contaminants and which practices a "fast food" nutritional mentality.

These and other matters relevant to your nutritional needs are explained more fully in your Assist Report.

The Questionnaire

The *Mercury Toxicity Diagnosis and Nutritional Evaluation Questionnaire* is a five hundred question instrument which provides an overview of the patient's dietary and health lifestyle. Again, the questionnaire is obtained through your Patient Advisor. It is important that all questions be answered, and that the answers be based upon the patient's current health status. Comments and written out answers should be brief and to the point.

Data from the questionnaire becomes a part of your Assist Report. In addition, the responses are compared with Dr. Huggins' experience in working with thousands of patients. In this way patients not only receive appropriate comparative information, but also become part of an ever expanding body of research.

In summary, the required tests and procedures (detailed above) are:

- A "hair" analysis (trace mineral analysis).
- A urine-mercury analysis.
- A CBC/blood profile.
- Completion of a *Mercury Toxicity Diagnosis and Nutritional Evaluation Questionnaire.*

Again, your Patient Advisor will assist you in obtaining all necessary tests and procedures.

Step Five
Providing for Proper Serum Compatibility Testing

Proper Serum Compatibility testing is actually one of the required laboratoray tests for both the In-Office and the Complete Assist programs.

It is essential that patients and health care practitioners assure themselves that the test results they receive are from either Huggins Diagnostic, Inc. or the affiliate laboratory, CompatLabs, Inc. Frankly, there are a great many testing formats offered by numerous individuals and organizations. Patients have occasionally contacted our office with reports from these unacceptable tests and we have found such test results unreliable for our work.

The serum compatibility test analyzes the patient's properly drawn blood specimen for the presence of antibodies. Antibodies indicate the materials which have already caused an adverse response within the patient.

This is a critical determination. Obviously, if you have already shown reactivity to a substance, you will not want that substance used in your replacement dental material. The important thing to note here is that *no one dental material is "safe" (non-reactive) for all patients.*

In line with this, the selection of your replacement dental material can be compared to buying a new suit of clothes. No one size, style, and color works for all people. You've got to get the right fit. Again, this is the situation with dental materials. Serum compatibility testing helps minimize the risk of replacing your amalgams with material which may also be unacceptable to your body.

Again, a word of caution is in order at this point concerning other types of "compatibility" tests. These other types of tests include illicit versions of serum compatibility testing, allergy testing, kinesiology, dermatron or vega machine testing, RAST testing, cytotoxic testing, voltmeter testing, electro acupuncture, reflexology, kevalite, barley green or pendulum testing. *None* of these forms of testing is an acceptable replacement to serum compatibility testing in Dr. Huggins' protocol.

Further, the patient is strongly encouraged to request verification from the doctor that the test results are actually from either Huggins Diagnostic, Inc. or its affiliate laboratory, CompatLabs, Inc. Both of these laboratories are Clinical Laboratories Improvement Act (CLIA) licensed facilities and perform serum compatibility testing according to Dr. Huggins' exacting specifications. No other test is accepted for Dr. Huggins' protocol.

Serum compatibility testing is easily obtained by contacting your patient advisor (800-331-2303). The test is available to health care practitioners around the world and may be ordered by your doctor. Specimens are drawn, frozen and shipped by overnight mail to either Huggins Diagnostic, Inc. (2535 Airport Rd., Colorado Srings, CO 80910) or CompatLabs, Inc. (1705 S. 8th St., Suite D, Colorado Springs, CO 80906).

Specially prepared kits are recommended for serum compatibility testing. These may also be ordered by contacting your Patient Advisor.

Five

Dental Care

Step Six
Preparing for Adequate Dental Care

Not all dentists are alike.

Most are unaware of the inherent dangers of amalgam toxicity, incompatibility of dental materials, or oral galvanic (electrical) impact from dissimilar metals placed in the mouth. Many who are aware of these factors have not been trained by Dr. Huggins, and even some who have attended one of Dr. Huggins' courses deviate from the required protocol.

If you choose to operate with our office "at a distance," your Patient Advisor will provide you with the names of those dentists closest to your location who are likely to practice the required protocol. It is necessary to emphasize, however, that each dentist is independent of Huggins Diagnostic Center. Accordingly, each dentist chooses what steps and procedures to include or omit in caring for his or her patients.

Your Patient Advisor will help you to know the steps in the accepted protocol, and you in turn will be able to discuss these matters with your dentist.

Again, dentists who practice the accepted protocol will incorporate the following into their treatment plan:

• The book *It's All in Your Head* as a basis for patient education.

- The required laboratory tests as a basis for the Assist Report.
- The Assist Report as a basis for individualized nutritional counseling and as a basis for specific supplementation.
- The Serum Compatibility test as a basis for recommending replacement dental materials.
- The sequential removal of fillings based upon electrical testing with an appropriate meter.
- The scheduling of dental appointments with appropriate consideration for patient immune cycles.
- The use of an air filtration system and/or an ion filtration (electrophoresis) system specifically designed to trap heavy metal contaminants such as mercury.
- The use of a rubber dam (where possible) during the dental procedures.

The first four recommendations have already been discussed previously. The others have not and, accordingly, information on these subjects now follows.

Sequential Removal:
Background of the Problem

Whenever two dissimilar metals are placed together, the potential for generating electric current arises. This fact is a basic truth taught in beginning chemistry courses. In addition it is a widely recognized (and carefully planned for) phenomenon in electrical engineering.

Dentistry has been aware of oral electrical possibilities from at least 1878. Consequently, articles published in national dental journals in the late 1800s and early 1900s cautioned against the use of dissimilar re-

storative metals. Again, it would appear that the practical aspects of less expensive dental materials which
were easier to use won out over these concerns. As a
result, the use of the amalgam became even more
widespread.

The standard amalgam filling contains mercury, silver, copper, tin, and zinc—five obviously dissimilar
metals. The potential for electric current is contained
when these dissimilar metals come together. This potential can then be activated by saliva within the mouth
which serves as an excellent electrolyte (a non-metallic
electric conductor). In addition, this "battery" within
your mouth is further activated by interaction with
other metallic restorations like nickel and gold crowns.

But how much current is generated?

The usual range of electric current generated by
fillings is from 2–3 microamps up to 100–200 microamps. Of course, a microamp is only a millionth of an
amp, and consequently this amount of current may not
seem like much.

The brain and human nervous system, however,
operate on a few billionths of an amp (nanoamps) of
current. In other words, the current generated by a
filling in your mouth is from 1,000–100,000 times
greater than that which operates your brain and nervous system.

Anyone who has had a toothache is well acquainted
with the fact that the nerves of your teeth relay to the
brain. It's all "wired" together.

Now, imagine your house.

What do you suppose would happen if you ran a
current through the wiring system of your home
100,000 times greater than that current on which it was
designed to function?

This may explain why some patients suffering from

multiple sclerosis and other neuro disorders have shown "miraculous" recoveries after the removal of their metallic fillings. Possibly, the electrical interference was the cause of the symptoms, and—when the source of the electrical interference was removed—the symptoms subsided.

Sequential Removal:
The Procedure to Apply

The problem of electrical current generated by metallic fillings is not always solved by simply removing the fillings. Dr. Huggins has discovered that fillings generate either negative or positive current. For some patients, removal of the positive fillings before removal of the negative fillings appears to permanently and destructively alter that patient's chemistry.

In addition, the strength of the current must also be considered.

Generally, Dr. Huggins recommends as an acceptable approximation the removal of amalgam filings on a quadrant by quadrant basis. The quadrant with the single highest negative fillings is removed first; then the quadrant with the next single highest negative until all quadrants with negative readings are removed. After the negative quadrants, the quadrant with the single highest positive reading is then removed. The quadrant with the next highest positive reading is then removed until all quadrants with positive readings have been replaced.

Again, the quadrant by quadrant approach is an approximation. Ideally (and for patients whose health is very serious), amalgam removal should be performed on a tooth by tooth basis throughout the entire mouth.

Also, when using the quadrant by quadrant approach, fillings within each individual quadrant should be removed from the highest negative to the lowest negative. Then—when all the negative fillings within that quadrant have been removed—the highest positive filling to the lowest positive filling should be replaced.

Sequential Removal:
Electrical Readings

Electrical readings using specifically identified micro-ammeters are reported in the Journal of the American Dental Association as far back as 1936. These meters were essentially the same as those used today.

Beyond this, Dr. Huggins recommends that the electrical reading be performed only once before, or at the same time as, *each* amalgam removal appointment. Metallic restorations discharge (like capacitors) after each reading. In addition, the current generated by fillings is not "fixed" over any appreciable period of time. Consequently, electrical readings should be performed once before each dental visit and the sequential removal guidelines modified as needed before the performance of each session's dental procedures.

A final practical note on sequential removal is in order. If the patient's health is not serious, it is usually more comfortable for the patient to have her or his dental work performed over two to three weeks (assuming numerous fillings). This allows the patient's gums to heal, and makes the entire dental process a more pleasant experience. Of course, for serious or urgent cases the dentistry can usually be performed over the course of a few days.

Root Canals

One of the most difficult decisions encountered by Dr. Huggins has been deciding that the removal of a tooth is frequently better for the patient than the possible problems which can be generated by a root canal. The metallic point of root canals appears to create a "lightning rod" effect and helps precipitate mercury from amalgams at the root tip.

Another concern is that clinical evidence indicates an autoimmune response may take place with root canals, regardless of the material used. The fact that the root canal filled tooth is essentially "dead" may trigger this response.

Gutta percha, a popular root canal material, actually contains aluminum and mercury. Consequently, gutta percha is undesirable. Beyond this, Dr. Huggins has reported difficulty in balancing the body chemistry of patients who have root canals.

Non-Precious Metals

Nickel crowns are common in dentistry. But most people (and even some dentists) are unaware that stainless steel dental appliances are made out of nickel alloy.

Unfortunately, nickel is a potential cancer producing agent. In addition, nickel—like other metals in the mouth—is a candidate for oral electrical phenomenon. As a result, consideration should be given to replacement of nickel restorations.

Composites

Again, it should be emphasized that no one dental material is non-reactive for all patients. Dental materials—including composites—should be selected on a case by case basis after serum compatibility testing. This is especially critical since many composites contain aluminum and/or tin. Both of these materials are heavy metal contaminants and may be harmful to the patient.

Consequently, certain composites may be unacceptable for the patient, and possible replacement of even these materials may need to be considered.

Patient Immune Cycles

Dr. Huggins has discovered that patient immune systems appear to function on twenty-one day cycles. These twenty-one day cycles—once started—can build upon each other until the immune system is significantly weakened. Obviously, penetrating mouth tissue with needles or clamps and drilling or removing teeth is an affront to the immune system. Consequently, scheduling dental work on the same day of the week over a period of several weeks can weaken the immune system and reduce the patient's ability to combat future exposure to disease.

Dental work should *not* be scheduled over a period of several weeks on the same day of the week. Rather, alternate days of the week (i.e., Monday for the first visit, Thursday for the second appointment, Tuesday for the third session, and Friday for the fourth visit) should be utilized in scheduling dental procedures.

Air and Ion Filtration Systems

The mercury vapor level in dental offices is generally magnitudes greater than the levels in ordinary air. This is true even in offices where amalgam is not placed, but only removed.

Consequently, Dr. Huggins recommends the use of either an air or an ion filtration system specifically designed to trap mercury vapor. Information on both of these systems is available from Huggins Diagnostic Center.

The key thing for the patient is that such a system should be in place in the dentist's office before dental procedures are performed.

Rubber Dams

The removal of amalgam generates mercury vapor and amalgam particles. Some of these particles are only dust, others are small "chunks."

The use of a properly placed rubber dam can help minimize the likelihood that these particles will be swallowed by the patient during the amalgam removal process.

Six

Follow-Up

Step Seven
Plan for Follow-Up or Comparison Testing

If you've ever listened to a discussion on major league batting, you've heard about the importance of follow-through on the swing. Failure to follow through is measured in lost hitting distance and in ineffective batting.

In the required protocol, "follow-up" is the same as follow-through in baseball.

Patient chemistries tend to vary after amalgam removal and further dietary and/or supplementation modification may be in order. As a result, Dr. Huggins recommends follow-up or recall testing for both In-Office and Complete Assist patients.

Your Patient Advisor will help you coordinate these follow-up reviews. Again, the required tests are listed below:

- A preliminary comparison or follow-up blood and urine test at three weeks to three months after amalgam removal.
- A second follow-up to include blood, hair, and urine tests at six months after the preliminary follow-up or comparison.
- Subsequent follow-up blood, hair, and urine tests at six months as required by your health needs.

Seven

Final Considerations

Sell Your Shotgun

American culture is inundated with the philosophy that "if a little is good, a lot is better." And this is the approach that most people take to vitamins and food supplements.

The problem here is that of imbalance.

The key to good health is a balanced chemistry. A balanced chemistry has enough of the right building materials in the proper proportion to each other. Simply consuming multitudes of different minerals and vitamins may actually do more harm than good.

An example of this is that of the canoe in a river. When a canoe rocks to one side people inside will sometimes throw themselves to the opposite side in an effort to overcome the rocking motion. However, the sudden shifting of weight within the canoe may actually capsize it due to the "imbalance" that has been created. As a result, instead of helping, the shifting of weight can hinder.

Supplementation can be like the canoe example. It is possible in this situation to take a portion of your chemistry that is essentially in appropriate relation to the rest of your body's needs and "imbalance" it.

Supplementation should be based on the specific needs of the patient as revealed by body chemistry analysis. This is why the Assist Report and the basic laboratory tests upon which it is based are key parts of the required protocol. Again, the Assist Report provides an analysis of the patient's individual needs and makes specific supplementation recommendations based on the patient's chemistries.

The Assist Report overcomes the "shotgun" mentality of overdosing a variety of supplements (potentially causing chemistry imbalances) in an effort to manage health problems. Instead, the patient is allowed to become a "sharpshooter" through the recommendation of specific supplements for specific needs.

Not All Supplements Are Created Equal

The Assist Report recommends the use of supplements from Matrix Minerals, Inc. (ordering information is available through your Patient Advisor). These supplements are specifically based upon Dr. Huggins' research and protocol. They reflect his exacting standards concerning quality and type of ingredients as well as supplementation dosage.

The patient needs to know that not all supplements are created equal.

Many supplements on the market today are made with biologically "non-active" materials. In other words, the supplement is not in a form that is usable or as usable to your body as another material would be. Examples of this are dolomite and oyster shell as calcium supplements. These forms of calcium are not as usable to your body as those used in the Matrix supplements.

It is important to know that there are three functions necessary to successfully balance the mineral requirements of the body. These are:

1. Absorption.
2. Distribution to the tissues.
3. Elimination of excess minerals.

Distribution is controlled by the heart and vascular system while elimination is directed by the liver and kidneys. Of course, neither distribution nor elimination are even at issue if the material is not first absorbed. And absorption is influenced by a multitude of factors.

Absorption factors include the mineral's form, the composition of the material enclosing it, the acidity of the stomach and intestine, and the body's actual need for that particular mineral. Since proper distribution and elimination are dependent upon the material being absorbed, the Matrix formulations emphasize maximum routes of absorption.

Accordingly, Matrix products are created by selecting the proper combination of minerals and then developing a "matrix" (multiple means of absorption). This "matrix" includes proteinates, chelates, ascorbates, citrates and other select acid ligands in a carbohydrate base.

This insures that the patient taking the Matrix product will receive greater opportunities within their own body chemistry of actually absorbing the supplement. It is important to keep this in mind since many food supplements on the market only allow one, rather than multiple, routes of absorption.

The old adage that "you get what you pay for" holds true in food supplements. Again, not all supplements are created equal, and only the Matrix products are based upon Dr. Huggins' research and requirements.

Just Give Me a Pill

In view of the recommended follow-up procedures, patients frequently ask how long they must stay with specific supplementation and dietary modification. The answer to this is ultimately dependent upon their personal health and their health lifestyle.

It must be kept in mind that our nation is a people of fast-food addicts. We are constantly bombarded with pollutants within and without our bodies. The nutritional value of most of our foods is "supplemented" with "vitamins" of questionable value.

Worse yet, because this is the environment we have grown up in, we like it this way.

We like the gooey, sugary, chocolatey pastries and candy bars with their refined carbohydrates, cadmium content, and especially their sugar. We are addicted to food deep fried at fast food stands in oil that has not been completely replaced every two hours and is full of free radicals. We can't live without soft drinks which are contaminated with aluminum (from the cans), sodium benzoate, [sugar substitutes] and other questionable "additives."

And when our health fails we want a pill that will make us better and allow us to continue to live our destructive health lifestyles.

How long do you have to change your lifestyle in order to be more healthy?

If you're a typical American, the answer is for the rest of your life.

Your supplementation regimen should change, however, as you modify your dietary lifestyle. Frankly, though, some degree of supplementation will probably always be advisable in order to maintain an optimal health level.

The key to all of this, however, is your personal commitment to change your life for the better. Ultimately, you are going to need motivation to do this.

The following incident sheds light on the kind of resolve it takes to change your health lifestyle for good:

A group of city commissioners was on a bus tour for the purpose of evaluating the problems of a major city slum. One of the commissioners, a woman, saw a five year old boy playing in a pile of rubble. The boy's clothes were tattered and torn, and the filth that was accumulated all over the boy's body and face had obviously been there for days.

The commissioner commented to the tour director, "That little boy's mother ought to at least clean him up!"

The tour director replied, "Commissioner, that little boy's mother probably loves him, but she doesn't hate dirt. You hate dirt, but you don't love that little boy enough to clean him up. . . . Until love for that little boy and hate for dirt are in the same person, that little boy will continue to be dirty."

Now, let's apply this observation to your health.

Do you want your health to be up to par? This alone probably won't be enough to permanently change your health lifestyle. Until the love of being healthy and *hate* for foods and habits that ruin your health exist within your person, you probably won't make a significant change in your way of living.

This scenario fits the condition of most Americans who "love" being healthy while at the same time they also "love" their destructive lifestyles. And so long as this is the case, the majority of people will continue to live with health that is below par. In the final analysis, many of these people actually want to continue living this way. If the option were available it's likely that they would choose to maintain their negative habits so long as they could "just take a pill" that would make them better.

However, the only available "pill" is constructive lifestyle change.

But now the good news: *you* don't have to be defeated by a destructive lifestyle.

You can choose to take the steps recommended in this book. You *really* can choose a PAR (proper amalgam removal) lifestyle.

This book has been written to inform people of their choice. And if you choose to make the recommended changes, then this book is dedicated to you.

Eight

How Root Canals Generate Toxins

"A new truth," warned Dr. Weston Price, "is like a new sense. You are now able to see things that you could not see before."

Dr. Weston Price, former director of research for the American Dental Association for 14 years, spent 35 years of his professional career researching the systemic diseases of the heart, kidney, uterus, nervous system and endocrine system that resulted from toxins seeping out of root canal filled teeth. A certain percentage of people are sensitive to toxins that are manufactured within these dead teeth.

Dr. Price saw many truths that even today we have a hard time seeing, for we are bogged down in "but we've always done it that way" thinking. We are too habitual to adopt his sense of "new truth." His observations led him far beyond the accepted remedies of that day. Incidentally, those remedies are basically the same treatments that are the foundation of today's root canal fundamentals. He researched 24 of those fundamentals and found each to be lacking.

Some of the "lacking" fundamentals included: X-rays revealing the presence of infection; infections expressing themselves as bone absorption; a given dental infection will express itself approximately the same in all people; if pus is flowing from a tooth it is a dangerous sign; and local comfort of a treated tooth is evidence of the success of a root filled tooth procedure.

He made quite a stir in the dental community. Even with his vast experience, educational background, and thousands of controlled experiments, dentists were resistant to changing their thinking about the root canal procedures that they had already been performing for decades.

What did Price find that convinced him that people could not tolerate root canals?

First he observed that if he removed root filled teeth from people suffering from kidney and heart disease, that in most cases, they would improve. In an effort to establish a relationship between the tooth and the disease, he inserted the root filled teeth under the skin of rabbits. Rabbits have a similar immune system to that of humans. In fact, a normal, non-infected human tooth (as removed for orthodontic reasons) can be inserted under the skin of a rabbit for a year with practically no reaction. A thin film will form over it, but microscopically there are no rejection cells present.

When a root filled tooth was implanted under the skin of a rabbit, the rabbit died within less than two days, sometimes within 12 hours. If a very small fragment (as an extract of the tooth) was used, within two weeks the rabbit would lose over 20% of its body weight, and die of heart disease if that is what the human donor had or kidney disease if that is what the human donor had. To further challenge this observation, he removed the fragment and transferred it to another rabbit. In two weeks he observed a duplicate performance. In one case, he reimplanted the same tooth fragment in 100 rabbits, each in succession dying from the same disease that the human had had. In most experimental cases he transferred the fragment 30 times.

As obvious as the consequences were, dentists persisted in placing root canal fillings. This, of course, caused a hot argument among dentists, and soon Dr. Percy R. Howe published a paper in the Journal of the National Dental Association rejecting Price's findings. Howe injected large amounts of the bacteria streptococcus into rabbits, and found no adverse reaction. This 1920 publication is still used as proof that root filled teeth are not harmful to humans.

In what way did Price show that Howe's paper was wrong?

In looking for a reason for the difference between Howe's findings and his own, Price investigated the methods of sterilization of root canals (similar to today's technology) and found that teeth retained their sterility for only about two days. Most lost sterility within less than 24 hours. Why? Where were these bacteria hiding? A tooth contains enamel, dentin, and a central pulp chamber. The central pulp chamber can be sterilized to a reasonable degree by removing its contents of nerves, arteries, and veins and flushing it with chemicals.

The dentin, however, is composed of thousands of tiny "dentin tubules" unreachable by this flushing procedure. Although microscopic in size, these tubules are quite adequate to house billions of bacteria. If one were to take a front tooth and arrange the dentin tubules end to end, they would reach for 3 miles. The tubules are wide enough to accommodate 8 streptococci abreast.

Where do these bacteria originally come from? They are of the streptococcus viridans family and are normal inhabitants of the mouth. When a tooth becomes decay prone, they invade the tooth and start killing tooth tissues. When they reach the pulp chamber, they invade not only the pulp tissue, but also the dentin tubules. When a dentist cleans out the pulp chamber, he removes all the bacteria in the chamber, but those bacteria that went into the tubules are still there. Then the dentist seals the tooth, and that's when a new truth begins that points out Howe's misinterpretation.

In an "anaerobic" condition, or one that contains no oxygen, these streptococci (specifically diploic and short chain strains) mutate, undergoing a slight change in body form and metabolism to adapt to this new environment. Now, instead of producing slightly offensive waste products, these transformed bacteria produce a potent poison called a toxin. Our immune system does not like the toxin, but the cells of our immune system cannot get in through the tiny holes in the outside of the root to destroy the bacteria. The toxins can seep out. Fluids containing nutrients can seep into the tooth, so the bacteria continue to thrive in confinement.

Howe's research addressed only the aerobic variety of bacteria, so completely missed the toxin-forming bacteria.

If the body launches a big fight against the toxins, then pus forms around the tooth. Conventional wisdom says that pus is bad for the patient, and we must give antibiotics until it is gone. Price found that pus was nearly sterile, and, though socially disagreeable, it's presence was a sign of successfully quarantining the toxins from the tooth. That was certainly a new idea, and not readily accepted as a "new truth."

Another upsetting situation pointed out by Price was that X-rays frequently miss abscesses that are on the front or back of a tooth. About 30% of the teeth have extra canals which may exit anywhere from half way down the tooth to all the way down at the tip like they are supposed to. They can exit on the front, back or side of the tooth. Those "other" canals that abscess are the ones that are apt to be missed on X-ray.

What about root filled teeth that do not form pus or give pain?

If the body's immune system is compromised, then very little action is initiated around the root filled tooth. Certain enzymes may escape which stimulate the bone to form what is termed "condensing osteitis" around the tooth. This is heavier than usual bone. It may actually fuse the surrounding bone to the tooth. On X-ray films, this will appear as a white line and is considered to reflect excellent healing. This tooth gives no trouble locally as far as pain and pus are concerned; but the toxins that seep out get into the circulation and with little immune system interference, seek a specific organ to attack. This Price called "tissue localization." Price had demonstrated this by transferring sections of root filled teeth from animal to animal, generating the same disease with each transfer.

What is the factor that determines who is most susceptible to having problems from root canals?

Price recorded 140,000 determinations in 1,200 patients to come up with his answer to this question. Bottom line, it is heredity. If your biological inheritance for two generations back, including brothers and sisters of your grandparents, were resistant to degenerative diseases, then you are of good stock. You are not apt to launch an immune response against a root canal. On the other hand, if there was a high frequency of heart, kidney, diabetes, reproductive disorders, etc., then you are more apt to be susceptible.

Sometimes a person of healthy genetic stock can develop diseases as a result of reactions to root filled teeth. How does this happen?

Most of us are aware that abuse of alcohol, drugs, and caffeine stresses our system. Price found that there were other stressors that were just as great. Exposure to these types of stressors tended to push people over their threshold and allow the root canal tooth to become a problem. The challenge could exceed the person's resistance.

He found that the two greatest stressors were pregnancy and influenza (the flu). Under the influence of either of these conditions, the toxins from root filled teeth were much more apt to produce disease at the person's specific susceptible site. Other stressors that upset root filled teeth were grief, anxiety, chilling, severe hunger, acute and chronic infection.

What if you have a root canal and want it removed? Do you just pull the tooth?

No, this might give more problems. When these teeth are removed, the attachment from the tooth to the bone called the periodontal ligament must be removed with a dental bur at the same time. This irritates the old bone, and stimulates it to form new bone. Recently in my studies at the University of Colorado where I was finishing a masters program in science, we were looking at biopsies of the bone under the root filled teeth that we had removed. The lymphocytes of autoimmune disease were embedded at least a millimeter into the bone, and sometimes more. All this must be removed if good bone healing is to be achieved.

Price's research, published in many peer reviewed journals (such as J.A.M.A., J.A.D.A.), has never been refuted. Commercial expediency has, no doubt, influenced the profession in its apparent decision to ignore this research (that of one of the most brilliant scientific

minds) to the detriment of an ever increasing proportion of the population.

Dr. Price, you certainly gave us a new insight with
your "new truth," and have given many of us dentists
cause for alarm. We must heed your advice and volu-
minous research, and set our personal prejudices
aside to consider your investigations. After all, it is the
quality of total life that is our concern, not just the
tooth, the whole tooth, and *nothing* but the tooth.

Nine

Cavitations

In the early 1950s, some European physicians and dentists noticed that certain old extraction sites had sealed over the top and a hole remained where the roots used to be. By the early 1960s, articles appeared in dental and medical journals in America describing Alveolar Cavitational Osteopathosis, or ACO (also called "cavitations" or "holes in the bone." These cavitations arose as a result of a lack of healing where the lining of the socket had not been removed.

Between the tooth and the bone there is a layer of connective tissue called the "periodontal ligament" ("perio" meaning "around," and "dontal" referring to the tooth). When a tooth is removed, that ligament most often remains behind. If it is not removed at the time of surgery, then the bone cannot regenerate to fill the space left behind. The socket will heal over with a thin layer of bone and new gum tissue, but the socket never fills in with good solid bone. As a result, there is a void or hole in the bone which is very unnatural and therefore this hole, the ligament and whatever toxins may be residing therein become a stress to the immune system.

This is demonstrated by viewing microscopic slides of the lining of the cavitations. A few, but very few, *streptococci* are found; but the notable finding is the presence of large, four-nuclei cells that are not readily identified as common cells (called "monocytes") that have left the bloodstream, grown and become what are called "tissue macrophages." These tissue macrophages (upon stimulation by chemicals somewhat specific to old extraction sites) subdivide their nuclei into four pieces. They can now process the tissue breakdown products.

These cells are definitely *not* the phagocytic polymorphonuclear leukocytes (PMNS) of infection fame. They represent more of an immunologic challenge.

When bone tissue biopsies have been performed on the bone immediately adjacent to a root canal-filled tooth, lymphocytic cells of chronic long-term immune challenge are frequently found in profusion. This is suggestive of a nidus of autoimmune disease. It also confirms the surgical recommendation of removing at least one millimeter of bone around the extraction site.

The sizes of the cavitations vary from a few millimeters to over a cubic centimeter and many patients have more than one. These are extremely difficult to see on x-ray and special training is necessary to identify and correct. Recently we have noted that in neurological diseases, the response of the patient can be quite dramatic immediately after a cavitation is properly treated.

The procedure to prevent cavitations from forming is very simple, fast and painless. Your dentist merely has to take an additional one minute after an extraction to clean out the socket with a slow speed drill and rinse it out properly. When this is done properly, the healing proceeds much more rapidly with much less bleeding or pain. You need a cavitation like you need another hole in your head.

Notes

CHAPTER ONE

1. Find a physician who has a Heidelberg Stomach Acid Test machine. Burning stomach sensations are not necessarily a sign of excessive stomach acid. They may also indicate an allergic food reaction, low stomach acid, Candida, or Campylobacter pyloritis. I strongly suggest that you take this medical test.
2. S. Itagaki, P. L. McGeer, and H. Akiyama, "Presence of T-Cytotoxic Suppressor and Leucocyte Common Antigen Positive Cells in Alzheimer's Disease Brain Tissue," *Neuroscience Letters* (October 1988):259–264.
3. The announcement was made by Dr. Henry Wisniewski of Senetek PLC in an article by United Press International published on June 26, 1986.
4. Dr. Gusella made this statement while appearing as a guest on the MacNeil/Lehrer News Hour on February 19, 1987.
5. See "Hydrocrabons," on page 56. I believe I "saw" my fingers leave my hand, and saw the floor in the spaces between, due to an extended separation of synapses caused by edema (swelling from fluid).
6. Marshall Mandell and Fran G. Mandell, *The Mandells' It's Not Your Fault You're Fat Diet* (New York: Plume, 1984).

7. Dr. Nasser made this statement during an address given in Tacoma, Washington, in March 1985.
8. Sam Ziff and Michael F. Ziff, *Infertility and Birth Defects: Is Mercury From Silver Dental Fillings an Unsuspected Cause?* (Orlando, Florida: Bio-Probe, 1987).
9. *Your Family Tree Connection*, by Chris M. Reading and Ross S. Meillon (New Canaan, Connecticut: Keats Publishing Inc., 1988), shows you how to shake your family tree for elusive clues to unlocking many diseases. Dr. Reading specializes in organic psychiatry, vitamin and mineral deficiencies, metabolic disorders, food allergies, clinical immunology/ecology, and genetics as they apply to neuropsychiatric disorders.
10. I now realize that the source of my mother's distress was very likely carbon monoxide from the leaky coal stove. Sometimes in the morning, my mother would look more dead than alive, her face chalk white.
11. I have learned since those years that the "poison" my mother feared could very well have been just that to her. The "dope" she protected herself from was the carbon monoxide from her coal stove, disagreeable ingredients in her favorite foods, chlorine in the water, lead from the old water pipes, and aluminum from her pitted aluminum pots and pans. All of these things can cause brain-fog reactions.
12. This is a prime example of why so many schizophrenic patients have such low self-esteem and try to keep off by themselves. Loneliness many times is a painful but preferable choice for them.
13. This was probably due to cerebral reactions to the welding fumes.
14. Formaldehyde and hydrocarbons in new books, mold in old books, and the heavy wax on school floors can cause both learning disabilities and inappropriate behavior in reactive, often highly intelligent students. If a student's handwriting becomes heavy or illegible, suspect brain allergies or Candida overgrowth. Read *An Alternative Approach to Allergies*, by Theron Randolph and Ralph W. Moss (New York: Lippincott and Crowell, Publishers, 1980); *Solving the Puzzle of the Hard to Raise Child*, by William G. Crook (New York: Random House, 1987); and *The Impossible Child in School, at Home: A Guide for Caring Teachers and Parents*, by Doris Rapp and Dorothy Bamberg (Tacoma, Washington: Practical Allergy Research Foundation, 1986). *The Impossible Child* should be required reading for teachers, child-welfare work-

ers, and the caring parents of troubled children for whenever the reason for their childrens' "impossible behavior" is not readily apparent.

15. I later learned that the sores on my face, neck, and arms were caused by mercury toxicity. They disappeared after all my silver fillings were removed a half-century later.

16. It was another decade before I learned that the ink in new textbooks and mold in old books can cause some students to suffer severe brain-fog reactions and to fall asleep in class.

I was once asked to help a student who was unable to complete his final examinations due to brain-fog reactions and flunked his courses. When I visited the student, I noticed that hundreds of books lined his bedroom walls. When I held a book near him, a whiff from it caused him to pass out for thirty minutes. When he awoke, he yelled, "What did you do?" I told him I suspected that books were the source of his distress, but he did not believe me. So rather than argue, I pushed the book back into his face again. He took another whiff and passed out for an additional twenty-five minutes. He removed the books from his sleeping area, and the following quarter, he earned straight A's.

Van Gogh's schizophrenia was probably caused by odors out-gassing from fresh paint. Many house painters also develop brain-fog reactions to paint fumes. Carpet layers react the same way to formaldehyde and other chemicals out-gassing from synthetic carpets. And many cooks react poorly to the gas fumes from their stoves and ovens.

CHAPTER TWO

1. Dr. Pleva was also a sufferer himself of the effects caused by silver amalgam fillings.

2. Dental detoxicologists, using a Mercury Vapor Analyzer, can easily determine if the amount of mercury escaping from amalgam fillings is toxic.

3. Patrick Störtebecker, M.D., former associate professor of neurology at the Karolinska Institute, Stockholm, Sweden, reports in his book *Mercury Poisoning From Dental Amalgam— A Hazard to the Human Brain* (Stockholm, Sweden: Störtebecker Foundation for Research, 1986) that the most dangerous injury caused by mercury vapor comes from mercury being absorbed from the upper nasal mucosa and passing

directly to the brain. He says, "Experimental findings have revealed that the brain accumulates about 10 times more mercury after exposure to mercury vapor, as compared to an equal amount of mercuric ions being injected or ingested."

4. According to Hal A. Huggins and Sharon A. Huggins in *It's All in Your Head* (Tacoma, Washington: Life Sciences Press, 1989), the acid environment and bacteria within the mouth cause mercury that leaches from silver fillings to combine with a carbon-hydrogen compound called a "methyl group." When mercury combines with a methyl group, it is called "methyl mercury." The process of combining is called "methylation."

5. Dr. Störtebecker also said, in a lecture entitled *Direct Transport of Mercury from the Oro-Nasal Cavity to the Cranial Cavity as a Cause of Dental Amalgam Poisoning*, given at Tufts University Dental School, Boston, on September 20, 1988, "Already 50 years ago Stock made an undeniable observation that inhaled mercury vapor spread to the mucosa of the upper nasal cavity directly to the brain."

6. About 100 years ago, mercury was used to block felt hats, which is where the phrase "mad as a hatter" originated.

7. I have noticed that mercury-sensitive individuals usually also develop acute allergic brain-fog reactions to chlorine.

8. *Neurology for Barefoot Doctors in All Countries: Correct Diagnosis by Simple Methods,* by Patrick Störtebecker (Stockholm, Sweden: Störtebecker Foundation for Research, 1988), should be required reading for every physician having anything to do with schizophrenic, Alzheimer's, or neurologically diseased patients. Another equally important book by Dr. Störtebecker is *Mercury Poisoning From Dental Amalgam— A Hazard to the Human Brain* (Stockholm, Sweden: Störtebecker Foundation for Research, 1986).

9. I had at least ten electrocardiograms due to premature ventricular contractions (PVCs) and chest pain, which disappeared after all the amalgam fragments were surgically removed from my gums and jawbone. Chest pain is a common phenomenon in mercury-toxic patients. It is possible that heart irregularities are caused by excessive electrical activity in the brain from metal in the oral cavity.

10. D. E. Vance, W. D. Ehmann, and W. R. Markesbery, "Trace Element Imbalances in Hair and Nails of Alzheimer's Disease Patients," *NeuroToxicology* 2 (1988):197–208.

11. This is according to *Direct Transport of Mercury from the Oro-Nasal Cavity to the Cranial Cavity as a Cause of Dental*

Amalgam Poisoning, a lecture given by Dr. Störtebecker at Tufts University Dental School, Boston, on September 20, 1988.

12. According to Charles H. Taft, a homeopathic dental surgeon, who presented a paper, *Injurious Effects of Amalgam Fillings, Medical Advance,* to the Massachusetts Dental Society on June 8, 1893. "I will simply quote from a patient from whom I removed some 25 amalgam fillings. . . . 'I had been under homeopathic treatment and for the first two years I experienced great relief, much better than ever before in my life, still the improvement was not as great and lasting as my physician had wished, and at his request I had all my fillings removed. . . . I can truly say I am glad it was done, my health has improved much faster since then and I have every reason to believe it was the mercury. . . . I now have better health than I have had for years, and it is steadily improving.'"

13. In January 1989, I met a scientist who, at one time, had worked for the National Aeronautics and Space Administration (NASA). He developed a computerized machine to diagnose diseases and to recommend their specific homeopathic remedies. After using the machine—which measures electrical activity at the fingertips—on me, he advised me to purchase seven homeopathic remedies.

    The following November, in Mexico, a man who was the fourth-generation homeopathic physician in his family advised me to buy four of the same remedies, three even matching the scientist's in strength. We only had a few minutes and did not have time to go any further, but he also told me that the higher levels of my brain were fine. My problem, he said, was with the transmission of my thought process at the nerve endings within my brain. He thought he could repair the damage within three to four months.

    It is important to understand that, at the time, all the metal had already been removed from my mouth.

14. I once met a naturopathic physician who looked into my eyes and diagnosed, in less than two minutes, the identical medical pathology that had taken many traditional physicians four years, at a cost of tens of thousands of dollars, to diagnose. In addition, he fixed a troublesome hiatal hernia in five minutes.

15. Panorex are like CAT scans of the teeth: the machine works its way around the head, starting at the back, to produce one long, complete shot of the whole jaw, instead of a series of separate shots of individual teeth.

16. Dr. Richard Glass, chairman and professor of oral pathology at the University of Oklahoma Health Science Center, reports that Candida yeast and other microorganisms have been found below the surface in dentures. He says that this type of Candida can cause the same problems associated with a regular Candida infection. If you suspect that Candida might be present in your dental plates, soak the plates overnight in a strong solution of Nystatin.

17. Ethylene diamine tetraacetic acid (EDTA) is a pharmaceutical drug that bonds (chelates) to heavy metals in the body, making them inactive and carrying them out of the body. It also stimulates the immune system and helps blood to flow easier by making platelets less sticky.

CHAPTER THREE

1. Stanley N. Wellborn, "Ordinary Electricity May Zap Your Health," *U.S. News and World Report* (date unknown).
2. I believe that physicians who prescribe antibiotics should tell their patients to take acidophilus or plain yogurt for ten days after the antibiotics are discontinued.
3. Dr. Denton is also considered to be the physician most informed in the United States about the connection between silver amalgam fillings and chronic disease.
4. D. E. Vance, W. D. Ehmann, and W. R. Markesbery, "Trace Element Imbalances in Hair and Nails of Alzheimer's Disease Patients, *NeuroToxicology* 2 (1988):197–208.

CHAPTER FOUR

1. I believe that all violent prisoners, depressed individuals, and hospitalized mental patients—as well as any disruptive people with an obnoxious personality—should refrain from using sugar in any form. They also should not use any white-flour products, food additives and colorings, cigarettes, chewing tobacco, chlorinated water, and chemicalized junk-food products. In addition, they should be tested for cerebral-allergic reactions to grains, milk, corn, soy-food colorings, monosodium glutamate (MSG), eggs, coffee, chlorine, formaldehyde, and hydrocarbons.
2. *Excessive* exercise can trigger reactions.

CHAPTER FIVE

1. The atrophy indicates that nutritional deficiencies are part of the pathology of the schizophrenia and Alzheimer's processes.

2. This is according to Dr. Hugh McDevitt, who was quoted by Shannon Browniee in her article, "The Body at War: Baring the Secrets of the Immune System," published in the July 2, 1990, issue of *U.S. News and World Report*.

3. William Backus and Marie Chapian, *Telling Yourself the Truth* (Minneapolis, Minnesota: Bethany House Publishers, 1980).

4. For more information on dysfunctional familial behavior and its effects, I recommend the following books: *The Dance of Anger*, by Harriet G. Lerner (New York: Harper and Row, 1985); *Men Who Hate Women and the Women Who Love Them*, by Susan Forward and Joan Torres (New York: Bantam Books, 1986); *Outgrowing the Pain*, by Eliana Gil (New York: Dell Publishing, 1988); and *Home Coming*, by John Bradshaw (New York: Bantam Books, 1990).

Glossary

Allergy. A negative reaction of body tissue to a specific substance.

Allopathic. Pertaining to any system of medical treatment using remedies that produce effects upon the body differing from those produced by disease; the opposite of "homeopathic."

Alzheimer's disease. A disease of the brain in which certain parts atrophy, causing a gradual deterioration of all brain function, which leads to psychosis and death.

Anatomic. Pertaining to the structural makeup of an organism or any of its parts.

Atrophy. A reduction in size of an organ, which in Alzheimer's disease is indicative of tissue degeneration of the brain; a wasting-away through lack of nutrition and use.

Brain fag. Brain fatigue.

Brain fog. Feeling of spaciness.

Carbon monoxide. A colorless, odorless, very toxic gas that burns to carbon dioxide with a blue flame and is formed as a product of the incomplete combustion of carbon.

Cerebrospinal. Pertaining to the cavities and canals of the brain and spinal cord.

Cerebrospinal fluid. The clear liquid surrounding the brain and spinal cord, and filling the cavities of the brain.

Chelation therapy. A type of treatment to remove unhealthy substances, such as metals and plaque, from the system. A chelating (bonding) agent, usually organic, is administered either orally or intravenously. It bonds with the metals or plaque, which are then excreted from the body along with it.

Clinical ecologist. An allergist who believes that the more symptoms a person has, both mental and physical, the more likely it is that he is suffering from an environmentally-induced disease.

Dental detoxicologist. A dentist who specializes in the *proper* removal and replacement of silver amalgam fillings and root canals.

Electroencephalogram. A graphic record of the minute changes in electrical activity of the cerebral cortex, as recorded by a machine called an "electroencephalograph."

Flatulence. Excess gas in the stomach or intestines.

Formaldehyde. A colorless, pungent, irritating, toxic gas made either by the oxidation of methanol or of gaseous hydrocarbons, and used chiefly as a disinfectant, a preservative, and a component in synthesizing many other compounds and resins.

Frontal lobe. The front of the brain; the part of the cerebral cortex in front of the central, and above the lateral, cerebral fissure.

Glutamic acid hydrochloric. An acid that converts to hydrochloric acid during the digestive process.

Homeopathy. The medical system that treats a disease or affliction using remedies producing effects similar to the suffering. Homeopathic physicians specialize in treating chronic disease.

Hydrocarbon. An organic compound, such as acetylene or benzene, containing only carbon and hydrogen, and often occurring in petroleum, natural gas, coal, and bitumens.

Hydrochloric acid. A normal acid in the stomach, comprised of hydrogen and chlorine, that digests proteins.

Iatrogenic. Pertaining to any disease that is doctor-induced through inappropriate treatment processes.

Immune system. The body's defense system against infection. It consists of the skin, the mucosa of the digestive tract, the digestive process itself, and the antibodies produced by the body.

Lesion. An abnormal change (wound or damage) in the structure of an organ or body part due to injury or disease, especially one that is circumscribed and well-defined.

Naturopathy. A therapeutic system that utilizes all of nature's agencies, forces, processes, and products, and avoids major surgery.

Neurology. The branch of medicine that focuses on the anatomy, physiology, and pathology of the nervous system.

Olfactory nerves. The sensory nerves that stretch from the olfactory bulb to the epithelial organs to facilitate the sense of smell.

Oncology. The scientific study of neoplastic (cancerous) growth.

Orthomolecular medicine. The branch of the study of nutrition that recognizes the individuality of each person, as well as the fact that some people require very large amounts of specific nutrients. It also takes into account that nutrients are often synergistic, with two or more working together to produce a specific effect.

Orthomolecular psychiatry. The branch of psychiatry that treats mental disorders by balancing the body's chemistry through vitamin, mineral, and nutritional therapy. Orthomolecular psychiatrists specialize in treating chronic, entrenched, long-standing schizophrenia after traditional treatment fails.

Pathology. The anatomic or physiologic deviations from the norm that constitute disease or characterize a particular disease.

Physianthropy. The study of the constitution of human beings, including diseases and their remedies.

Schizophrenia. A psychotic disorder characterized by a loss of contact with reality and the disintegration of the personality.

Septum. A partition of tissue that forms a dividing wall between two spaces or cavities.

Synergistic. Cooperative; working together.

Temporal lobe. The lobe in the brain located below the lateral cerebral fissure and continuous posteriorly with the occipital lobe.

Trace mineral. An element that is present in an organism in minute quantities but is essential to its life.

Venous system. As used in this book, the system of veins in the brain.

Ventricle. A small cavity or chamber in the body; one part of the system of communicating cavities within the brain that is continuous with the central canal of the spinal cord.

Bibliography

BOOKS

Airola, Paavo. *Are You Confused?* Phoenix, Arizona: Health Plus, Publishers, 1971.

Airola, Paavo. *How to Get Well*. Phoenix, Arizona: Health Plus, Publishers, 1974.

Backus, William, and Marie Chapian. *Telling Yourself the Truth*. Minneapolis, Minnesota: Bethany House Publishers, 1980.

Bieler, Henry G. *Food Is Your Best Medicine*. New York: Vantage Press, Inc., 1973.

Bircher-Benner, M. *Digestive Problems*. New York: Jove Publishers, 1978.

Blaine, Tom R. *Mental Health Through Nutrition*. Secaucus, New Jersey: Citadel Press, 1974.

Bland, Jeffrey. *Biochemical Aspects of Mental Illness*. Seattle, Washington: Well Mind Association, 1979.

Bland, Jeffrey. *Your Health Under Siege*. Brattlesboro, Vermont: Greene, 1982.

Bricklin, Mark. *Practical Encyclopedia of Natural Healing*. Emmaus, Pennsylvania: Rodale Press, 1983.

Busick, Bonnie S., and Martha Gorman. *Ill, Not Insane*. Boulder, Colorado: New Idea Press, Inc., 1986.

Cammer, Leonard. *Up From Depression*. New York: Pocket Books, 1976.

Chaitow, Leon. *Candida Albicans: Could Yeast Be Your Problem?* London: Thorsons, 1985.

Coca, Arthur F. *The Pulse Test.* New York: Arco, 1978.

Collison, David R. *Why Do I Feel So Awful?* London: Angus and Robertson Publishers, 1989.

Conn, Eric E., et al. *Outlines of Biochemistry.* New York: John Wiley and Sons Inc., 1963.

Crook, William G. *Solving the Puzzle of the Hard to Raise Child.* New York: Random House, 1987.

Crook, William G. *The Yeast Connection: A Medical Breakthrough.* Jackson, Tennessee: Professional Books, 1983.

Crook, William G., and Marjorie Hurt Jones. *The Yeast Connection Cookbook.* Jackson, Tennessee: Professional Books, 1989.

Dadd, Debra Lynn. *Nontoxic and Natural: How to Avoid Dangerous Everyday Products and Buy or Make Safe Ones.* New York: J. P. Tarcher, 1984.

Davis, Adelle. *Let's Get Well.* New York: Signet, 1972.

Davis, Adelle. *You Can Get Well.* Simi Valley, California: Poorboy Press, 1975.

Diamond, Harvey, and Marilyn Diamond. *Fit for Life.* New York: Warner Books, 1984.

Diamond, John. *Your Body Doesn't Lie.* New York: Warner Books, 1980.

Dufty, William. *Sugar Blues.* New York: Warner Books, 1986.

Foreman, Robert. *How to Control Your Allergies.* New York: Larchmont Books, 1979.

Fredericks, Carlton. *Nutrition Handbook.* Canoga Park, California: Major Books, 1976.

Fredericks, Carlton, and Herman Goodman. *Low Blood Sugar and You.* New York: Constellation International, 1976.

Gennaro, Alfonso R., ed. *Remington's Pharmaceutical Sciences.* Oradell, New Jersey: Medical Economics, 1985.

Hausman, Patricia. *The Right Dose.* Emmaus, Pennsylvania: Rodale Press, 1987.

Heritage, Ford. *Composition and Facts About Foods.* Mokelumne Hill, California: Health Research, 1971.

Hoffer, Abram. *Common Questions on Schizophrenia and Their Answers.* New Canaan, Connecticut: Keats Publishing Inc., 1987.

Hoffer, Abram. *Orthomolecular Medicine for Physicians.* New Canaan, Connecticut: Keats Publishing Inc., 1989.

Hoffer, Abram, and Morton Walker. *Nutrients to Age Without*

Senility. New Canaan, Connecticut: Keats Publishing Inc., 1980.

Hoffer, Abram, and Morton Walker. *Orthomolecular Nutrition.* New Canaan, Connecticut: Pivot Books, 1978.

Huggins, Hal A. *Why Raise Ugly Kids?* Westport, Connecticut: Arlington House Publications, 1981.

Huggins, Hal A., and Sharon A. Huggins. *It's All in Your Head.* Tacoma, Washington: Life Sciences Press, 1989.

Jordan, William H., Jr. *Windowsill Ecology.* Emmaus, Pennsylvania: Rodale Press, 1977.

Kenyon, Julian N. *Clinical Ecology: The Treatment of Ill Health Caused by Environmental Factors.* London: Thorsons, 1985.

Kirschmann, John D., and Lavon J. Dunne. *Nutrition Almanac.* New York: McGraw-Hill Publishing, 1984.

Krantz, John C., Jr., and C. Jelleff Carr. *Pharmacologic Principles of Medical Practice.* Baltimore, Maryland: Williams and Wilkins, 1961.

Kunin, Richard A. *Mega-Nutrition: The New Prescription for Maximum Health, Energy and Longevity.* New York: Signet, 1984.

Kushi, Michio, and the East West Foundation. *The Macrobiotic Approach to Cancer.* 2d ed. Garden City Park, New York: Avery Publishing Group, 1991.

LaFavore, Michael. *Radon: The Quiet Killer.* Emmaus, Pennsylvania: Rodale Press, 1987.

Leonard, Jon N., J. L. Hoffer, and N. Pritikin. *Live Longer Now.* New York: Grosset and Dunlap, 1977.

Lesser, Michael. *Nutrition and Vitamin Therapy.* Berkeley, California: Nutritional Medicine, 1985.

Lieberman, Shari, and Nancy Bruning. *The Real Vitamin and Mineral Book: Going Beyond the RDA for Optimum Health.* Garden City Park, New York: Avery Publishing Group, 1990.

MacKarness, Richard. *Chemical Victims.* London: Pan Limited, 1980.

Mandell, Fran G. *Dr. Mandell's Allergy-Free Cookbook.* New York: Pocket Books, 1981.

Mandell, Marshall. *Dr. Mandell's Lifetime Arthritis Relief System.* New York: Coward, McCann, 1983.

Mandell, Marshall, and Fran G. Mandell. *The Mandells' It's Not Your Fault You're Fat Diet.* New York: Plume, 1984.

Mandell, Marshall, and Lynne Waller Scanlon. *Dr. Mandell's 5-Day Allergy Relief System.* New York: Pocket Books, 1980.

Manning, Betsy Russell. *Candida, Silver (Mercury) Fillings and the Immune System*. San Francisco: Greensward Press, 1990.

McDougall, John A., and Mary A. McDougall. *The McDougall Plan*. Piscataway, New Jersey: New Century, 1983.

Mindell, Earl. *Unsafe at Any Meal*. New York: Warner Books, 1987.

Mindell, Earl. *Vitamin Bible*. New York: Warner Books, 1981.

Morgan, Brian, and Roberta Morgan. *Brainfood: Nutrition and Your Brain*. Tucson, Arizona: The Body Press, 1987.

Padus, Emrika. *The Complete Guide to Your Emotions and Your Health: New Dimensions in Mind-Body Healing*. Emmaus, Pennsylvania: Rodale Press, 1986.

Pelton, Ross. *Mind, Food and Smart Pills*. Los Angeles: T. R. Publishing, 1986.

Pfeiffer, Carl C. *Mental and Elemental Nutrients: A Physician's Guide to Nutrition and Health Care*. New Canaan, Connecticut: Keats Publishing Inc., 1975.

Pfeiffer, Carl C. *Nutrition and Mental Illness*. Rochester, Vermont: Healing Arts Press, 1987.

Philpott, William H., and Dwight K. Kalita. *Brain Allergies: The Psychonutrient Connection*. New Canaan, Connecticut: Keats Publishing Inc., 1980.

Physician's Desk Reference. Oradell, New Jersey: Medical Economics, 1991.

Pottenger, Frances F. *Pottenger's Cats*. La Mesa, California: Price-Pottenger Foundation, 1983.

Prevention Magazine Editors. *The Complete Book of Vitamins and Minerals for Health*. Emmaus, Pennsylvania: Rodale Press, 1984.

Prevention Magazine Editors. *Fighting Disease*. Emmaus, Pennsylvania: Rodale Press, 1984.

Prevention Magazine Editors. *Future Youth: How to Reverse the Aging Process*. Emmaus, Pennsylvania: Rodale Press, 1987.

Prevention Magazine Editors. *Understanding Vitamins and Minerals*. Emmaus, Pennsylvania: Rodale Press, 1984.

Prevention Magazine Editors and Sharon Faelten. *The Allergy Self Help Book: A Complete Guide to Detection and Natural Treatment of Allergies*. Emmaus, Pennsylvania: Rodale Press, 1986.

Prevention Magazine Editors and Sharon Faelten. *Minerals for Health*. Emmaus, Pennsylvania: Rodale Press, 1981.

Randolph, Theron G. *Human Ecology and Susceptibility to the*

Chemical Environment. Springfield, Illinois: Charles C. Thomas Publishers, 1978.

Randolph, Theron G., and Ralph W. Moss. *An Alternative Approach to Allergies.* New York: Lippincott and Crowell, Publishers, 1980.

Randolph, Theron G., and Dorothy C. Weidman. *The Realities of Food Addiction: Discharge Instructions for Hospitalized Patients.* Chicago: Human Ecology Action League (HEAL), 1984.

Rapp, Doris. *Allergies and the Hyperactive Child.* New York: Fireside, 1985.

Rapp, Doris, and Dorothy L. Bamberg. *The Impossible Child in School, at Home: A Guide for Caring Teachers and Parents.* Tacoma, Washington: Practical Allergy Research Foundation, 1986.

Reading, Chris M., and Ross S. Meillon. *Your Family Tree Connection.* New Canaan, Connecticut: Keats Publishing Inc., 1988.

Reuben, David. *Everything You Always Wanted to Know About Nutrition.* New York: Avon Books, 1979.

Rinkel, H. J., T. G. Randolph, and M. Zeller. *Food Allergy.* Norwalk, Connecticut: New England Foundation of Allergic and Environmental Diseases, 1951.

Salaman, Maureen. *Nutrition: The Cancer Answer.* Statford, California: Statford Publishing Inc., 1989.

Sattilaro, Anthony J., and Tom Monte. *Recalled by Life.* New York: Avon Books, 1982.

Schauss, Alexander G. *Diet, Crime, and Delinquency.* Tacoma, Washington: Life Sciences Press, 1988.

Sheinkin, David, et al. *Food, Mind and Mood.* New York: Warner Books, 1979.

Simonton, Carl O., et al. *Getting Well Again.* New York: Bantam Books, 1981.

Siskind, Linda. *The Pesticide Syndrome.* San Francisco: Earthwork Publications, 1979.

Smith, Lendon. *Feed Your Kids Right.* New York: Dell Publishing, 1984.

Smith, Lendon. *Feed Yourself Right.* New York: Dell Publishing, 1985.

Störtebecker, Patrick. *Dental Caries as a Cause of Nervous Disorders.* Stockholm, Sweden: Störtebecker Foundation for Research, 1986.

Störtebecker, Patrick. *Mercury Poisoning From Dental Amal-*

gam—A Hazard to the Human Brain. Stockholm, Sweden: Störtebecker Foundation for Research, 1986.

Störtebecker, Patrick. *Neurology for Barefoot Doctors in All Countries: Correct Diagnosis by Simple Methods.* Stockholm, Sweden: Störtebecker Foundation for Research, 1988.

Trowbridge, John Parks, and Morton Walker. *The Yeast Syndrome.* New York: Bantam Books, 1986.

Truss, C. Orian. *The Missing Diagnosis.* Birmingham, Alabama: C. Orian Truss, 1983.

Vithoulkas, George. *Homeopathy: Medicine of the New Man.* New York: Arco, 1979.

Walker, N. W. *Raw Vegetable Juices.* New York: Jove Publishers, 1977.

White, Kristin. *Diet and Cancer.* New York: Bantam Books, 1984.

Williams, Roger. *Nutrition Against Disease.* New York: Bantam Books, 1973.

Wright, Jonathan V. *Healing With Nutrition.* Emmaus, Pennsylvania: Rodale Press, 1984.

Wunderlich, Ray C., Jr., and Dwight K. Kalita. *Candida Albicans.* New Canaan, Connecticut: Keats Publishing Inc., 1984.

Ziff, Sam. *Silver Dental Fillings: The Toxic Time Bomb.* New York: Aurora Press, 1984.

Ziff, Sam, and Michael F. Ziff. *Infertility and Birth Defects: Is Mercury From Silver Dental Fillings an Unsuspected Cause?* Orlando, Florida: Bio-Probe, 1987.

Ziff, Sam, and Michael F. Ziff. *Mercury Detoxification.* Orlando, Florida: Bio-Probe, 1988.

ARTICLES AND RESEARCH PAPERS

Abraham, J. E., C. W. Svare, and C. W. Frank. *The Effect of Dental Amalgam Restorations on Blood Mercury Levels.* Iowa City, Iowa: University of Iowa College of Medicine, 1983.

Aldous, Jay A., G. Lynn Powell, and Suzanne S. Stensaas. "Brain Abscess of Odontogenic Origin: Report of a Case." *JADA Journal* (December 1987).

Anderson, Nancy C. "Brave New World." *Vogue* (January 1990).

Appel, Stanley H. "A Unifying Hypothesis for the Cause of Amyotrophic Lateral Sclerosis, Parkinsonism, and Alzheimer's Disease." In *Neurological Progress,* ed. American Neurological Association.

Bird, Christopher. "Gaston Naessens: Discoverer of the Somatid." *Health Consciousness* (December 1990).

Boucher, Louis J., ed. "Quantization of Nickel and Beryllium Leakage from Base Metal Casting Alloys." *Journal of Prosthetic Dentistry* (July 1985):127–135.

Browniee, Shannon. "The Body at War: Baring the Secrets of the Immune System." *U.S. News and World Report* (2 July 1990).

Campbell, Stephen D., Edwin J. Riley, and Ralph B. Sozio. "Evaluation of a New Epoxy Resin Die Material." *Journal of Prosthetic Dentistry* (July 1985).

Cooper, G. P., and R. S. Manalis. "Influence of Heavy Metals on Synaptic Transmission: A Review." *NeuroToxicology* (1983).

Djerassi, E., and N. Berova. "The Possibilities of Allergic Reactions From Silver Amalgam Restorations." *International Dentistry Journal* (1969):481–488.

Drake, Miles E., Jr. "The Association of Motor Neuron Disease and Alzheimer-Type Dementia." *American Journal of Medical Sciences* (1984).

Dwivedi, Chandradhar, et al. "Effect of Mercury Compounds on Cholineacetyl Transferase." *Research Communications in Chemical Pathology and Pharmacology* (November 1980):381–384.

Ehler, S. F. "The Assessment of Mercury in Mouth Air." *Journal of Dental Research,* Special Issue, Abstracts (March 1985):652.

Ehmann, W. D., W. R. Markesbery, M. Alauddin, T.I.M. Hossain, and E. H. Brubaker. "Brain Trace Elements in Alzheimer's Disease." *New Toxicology* 7 (1986):197–206.

Findlay, Steven, and Shannon Browniee. "The Delicate Dance of the Body and Mind." *U.S. News and World Report* (2 July 1990).

Fredericks, Carlton. "Organized Dentistry's Poisonality." *Let's Live* (February 1988).

Friberg, Lars, Leif Kullman, Birger Lind, and Magnus Nylander. "Mercury in the Central Nervous System in Relation to Amalgam Fillings." *Lakartidningen* (1986):519–522.

Guyer, Samuel, William Lefkowitz, William F. P. Malone, John E. Rhoads, and Robert C. Sproull. "Biocompatability of Base Metal Alloys." *Journal of Prosthetic Dentistry* (July 1987):1–5.

Guyer, Samuel, William Lefkowitz, William F. P. Malone, John E. Rhoads, and Robert C. Sproull. "Effect of Dental Amalgam and Nickel Alloys on T-Lymphocytes: Preliminary Report." *Journal of Prosthetic Dentistry* (May 1984):617–625.

Hahn, Leszek J., Reinhard Kloiber, Murray J. Vimy, Yoshimi Takahashi, and Fritz L. Lorscheider. *Dental "Silver" Tooth Fillings: A Source of Mercury Exposure Revealed by Whole-*

Body Image Scan and Tissue Exposure. Calgary, Alberta, Canada: Faculty of Medicine, University of Calgary, August 1989.

Hanson, Mats. "Effects of Inorganic Mercury on the Nervous System." *Bio-Probe* (March 1988).

Hornykiewicz, Oleh, and Stephen J. Kish. "Neurochemical Basis of Dementia in Parkinson's Disease." *Journal Canadien des Physiologie et Pharmacologie* (February 1984).

Itagaki, S., P. L. McGeer, and H. Akiyama. "Presence of T-Cytotoxic Suppressor and Leucocyte Common Antigen Positive Cells in Alzheimer's Disease Brain Tissue." *Neuroscience Letters* (October 1988):259–264.

Komulainen, Hannu, and Jouko Tuomisto. "Effect of Heavy Metals on Dopamine, Noradrenaline and Serotonin Uptake and Release in Rat Brain Synaptosomes." *Acta Pharmacol* (1981):199–204.

Kuntz, William D., Roy M. Pitkin, Albert W. Bostrom, and Mark S. Hughes. *Maternal and Cord Blood Background Mercury Levels: A Longitudinal Surveillance*. Iowa City, Iowa: University of Iowa College of Medicine, 1982.

Kupsinel, Roy. "Opthalmologist's Diagnosis: 'Optic Neuritis,' Final Diagnosis: Mercury Poisoning." *Health Consciousness* (1986):41–42.

Lamm, O., and H. Pratt. "Subclinical Effects of Exposure to Inorganic Mercury Revealed by Somatosensory-Evoked Potentials." *European Neurology* 24 (1985):237–243.

Langan, Dan C., P. L. Fan, and Alice A. Hoos. "The Use of Mercury in Dentistry: A Critical Review of the Recent Literature." *JADA Journal* (December 1987):867–880.

Malamud, Daniel, Scott A. Dietrich, and Irving M. Shapiro. "Low Levels of Mercury Inhibit the Respiratory Burst in Human Polymorphonuclear Leukocytes." *Biochemical and Biophysical Research Communications* (16 May 1985):1145–1151.

McGeer, P. L., et al. "Aging, Alzheimer's Disease, and the Cholinergic System of the Basal Forebrain." *Neurology* (June 1984).

McGovern, J. J., Jr., et al. *Use of Phenylated Food Compounds in Diagnosis and Treatment of 100 Patients With Food Allergy and Phenol Intolerance*. Provo, Utah: Brigham Young University.

McKay, S. J., J. M. Reynolds, and W. J. Racz. "Differential Effects of Methylmercuric Chloride and Mercuri Chloride on the L-Glutamate and Potassium Evoked Release of (-H) Dopamine from Mouse Striatal Slices." *Canadian Journal of Physiology and Pharmacology* 64 (1986).

Miyamoto, Michael D. "Hg2+ Causes Neurotoxicity at an Intracellular Site Following Entry Through Na and Ca Channels." In *Brain Research,* ed. Elsevier Biomedical Press (1983).

Nadimi, Hasan, Andrew T. Bronny, Aldo Sbigoli, William M. Gatti, and Peter Hasiakos. "Aneurysmal Bone Cyst Associated With a Dentigerous Cyst: Report of Case." *JADA Journal* (December 1987).

"Noradrenaline, Serotonin and Their Metabolites in Parkinson's." *Brain Research* (1983):321–328.

Nylander, Magnus. "Mercury in Pituitary Glands of Dentists." *Lancet* 4025 c 22 JR-disc 6A.

Patterson, J. E., B. G. Weissberg, and P. J. Dennison. "Mercury in Human Growth from Dental Amalgams." In *Environmental Contamination and Toxicology,* ed. Chemistry Division, DSIR, Private Bag, Petone, New Zealand, and Dental Department, Porirua Hospital, Porirua, New Zealand (1985):459–468.

Raianna, B., and M. Hobson. "Influence of Mercury on Uptake of (3Hl Dopamine and I H) Norepinephrine by Rat Brain Synaptosomes." *Toxicology Letters* 25 (1985):7–14.

Reilly, David Taylor, et al. "Is Homeopathy a Placebo Response?" *Lancet* (1986).

Ruberg, Merle, et al. "Muscarinic Binding and Choline Acetyltransferase Activity in Parkinsonian Subjects With Reference to Dementia." *Brain Research* (1982).

Snapp, K. A., et al. "Contribution of Dental Amalgams to Blood Mercury Levels." *Journal of Dental Research,* Special Issue, Abstract 1276 (March 1986):311.

Svare, Carl W. "Dental Amalgam Related Mercury Vapor Exposure." *CDA Journal* (October 1984):54–60.

Utt, Harold D. "Mercury Breath . . . How Much Is Too Much?" *CDA Journal* (1984):41–45.

Vance, D. E., W. D. Ehmann, and W. R. Markesbery. "Trace Element Imbalances in Hair and Nails of Alzheimer's Disease Patients." *NeuroToxicology* 2 (1988):197–208.

Vasken, Aposhian H. "DMSA and DMPS—Water Soluble Antidotes for Heavy Metal Poisoning." *Pharmacol Toxicol* 23 (1983):193–215.

Verschaeve, L., M. Kirsch-Volders, C. Suzanne, C. Groetenbriel, R. Haustermans, A. Lecomte, and Roossels. "Genetic Damage Induced by Occupationally Low Mercury Exposure." *Environmental Research* (1976):306–316.

Vimy, M. J., and F. L. Lorscheider. "Intra-Oral Air Mercury Released From Dental Amalgam." *Journal of Dental Research* (August 1985):1069–1071.

Vimy, M. J., and F. L. Lorscheider. "Serial Measurements of Intra-Oral Air Mercury: Estimation of Daily Dose From Dental Amalgam." *Journal of Dental Research* (August 1985):1072–1075.

Vimy, M. J., A. J. Luft, and F. L. Lorscheider. "Estimation of Mercury Body Burden From Dental Amalgam: Computer Simulation of a Metabolic Compartmental Model." *Journal of Dental Research* (December 1986):1415–1419.

Vimy, M. J., Y. Takahashi, and F. L. Lorscheider. "Maternal-Fetal Distribution of Mercury (203-Hg) Released From Dental Amalgam Fillings." *American Physiological Society* (1990).

Wellborn, Stanley N. "Ordinary Electricity May Zap Your Health." *U.S. News and World Report* (date unknown).

Wolfe, Bill, and Penny Davis Wolfe. "Fillings, Mercury and You." *Mothering* (Summer 1987).

Wolff, Mark, John W. Osborne, and Albert L. Hanson. "Mercury Toxicity and Dental Amalgam." *NeuroToxicology* (1983):201–204.

Index

biocompatibility of
materials used in, 41,
43, 47
composite, 34, 43
copper, 45–46
galvanic reactions
caused by, 48–49
removal of, 40–45, 73,
94
resin, 46–47
silver. *See* Dental fillings, amalgam.
Dental fragments
in gums and jawbone,
36, 37, 41–42, 47
removal of, 3, 43
*Dental "Silver" Tooth
Fillings: A Source of
Mercury Exposure
Revealed by Whole-
body Image Scan and
Tissue Exposure,* 32–33
Denton, Sandra, 65
Dentures, 42–43
Depression, 62, 93,
104–105, 108
Detoxification of the body,
68–69
Diabetes, 3, 84–85, 87,
89–90, 109
Diamond, John, 6, 79
Diet
four-day rotation, 89,
91–92
high-complex-carbohy-
drate, 89, 90
importance of, 83–85,
108
low-carbohydrate, 62–
63, 87–89, 97
vegetarian, 90
Digestion, importance of,
13
Digestive enzymes, 63, 78

Dinoseb, 55
*Dr. Mandell's 5-Day
Allergy Relief System,*
5
*Dr. Mandell's Lifetime
Arthritis Relief System,*
6
Doyle, Arthur Conan, 51
Dufty, William, 108
Dysfunctional familial
behavior, 109–110

Eastern State Hospital, 24
Electric Power Research
Institute, 58
Electricity, within the
body, 48–49. *See also*
Electrolytes.
Electroencephalogram, 23
Electrolytes, 97–98
Electromagnetic fields,
58–59
Ely, John T. A., 103
Ely, Thomas, 31
Environmental Protection
Agency, 29, 38, 56, 59
Epilepsy, 49
Ethylene diamine
tetraacedic acid
(EDTA), 47
Exercise, 92–93, 108, 109

Facts and Comparisons,
94
Fat
body, 68–69
in the diet, 84–85
Feed Yourself Right, 5, 79
Fighting Disease, 79
Filters
air, 62
water, 60, 105
Findlay, Steven, 102
Folic acid, 36, 75, 79, 106